Let Your Light Shine Through

Strategies for Living With Myalgic Encephalomyelitis/ Chronic Fatigue Syndrome, Fibromyalgia and Multiple Chemical Sensitivity

Eleanor Stein, MD, FRCP(C)

ISBN 978-0-9881510-2-4

Second Edition, 2025

Praise for Let Your Light Shine Through

In *Let Your Light Shine Through*, Dr. Ellie Stein has distilled her own lived experience, her years of caring for people with ME/CFS and similar illness, and her training as a psychiatrist into incredibly helpful, practical suggestions for dealing with these complex disorders. The manual gives patients and their caregivers ideas on how to manage their energy and day-to-day symptoms, including pain, lightheadedness, and sleep disruption. It should be required reading for everyone who treats people with ME/CFS, FM and MCS, and I would add Long COVID as well. This is a superb resource!

Peter C. Rowe, MD
Professor of Pediatrics & Director, Chronic Fatigue Clinic
Johns Hopkins Children's Center

Dr. Eleanor Stein brings rare clarity to complex conditions like ME/CFS and long COVID. This thoughtful, grounded manual offers a flexible, nervous-system–informed framework that emphasizes self-observation over rigid rules. Compassionate, practical, and deeply credible, it's a steady guide for anyone seeking understanding, regulation, and forward movement without fear.

Raelan Agle, MSW — founder of the Brain Retraining 101 program, author, and YouTuber

Dr. Ellie Stein's book is an invaluable, accessible guide for people living with ME/CFS, fibromyalgia, long COVID, and military and civilian toxic injuries. Her practical self-management strategies empower patients to reduce relapses, increase day-to-day stability, and realize genuine clinical improvement. This well-structured, easy-to-follow resource transforms complex care into actionable steps, offering hope and tangible benefits to those striving for a more reliable and fulfilling life.

Nancy Klimas, MD, Director, Institute for Neuro Immune Medicine
Professor and Chair, Department of Clinical Immunology
Dr. Kiran Patel College of Osteopathic Medicine, Nova Southeastern University

A compassionate, science-based guide to living with ME/CFS, fibromyalgia, and MCS. Drawing on decades of clinical expertise and lived experience, Dr. Eleanor Stein offers practical, evidence-informed strategies that validate the challenges of chronic illness while guiding readers to make meaningful, sustainable steps toward better health.

James Davis
President, ME International

This is an essential resource for anyone treating or living with ME/CFS, fibromyalgia, or MCS. It deserves a place on the shelf of every integrative medicine practitioner and would benefit all physicians who encounter these often-misunderstood conditions. Most importantly, it offers patients a compassionate, realistic roadmap for managing their health and maximizing their quality of life.

Josh Helman, MD, Harvard-trained Physician, CMO of DrJosh.com

I strongly recommend *Let Your Light Shine Through* as a highly practical and well-structured resource for people living with ME/CFS and related complex chronic illnesses. This is a truly comprehensive workbook that will help readers better understand their symptom patterns and make informed, individualized decisions towards a better life.

Patrick Ussher, Author of Understanding ME/CFS & Strategies for Healing.

Let Your Light Shine Through reflects a career's worth of work by an exceptional physician. I regularly recommend this book and Dr. Stein's other resources to patients with complex chronic conditions. It is well organized, accessible, and allows patients to engage at their own pace.

Jennifer Swales, MBBS, CCFP
Staff Physician, Environmental Health Clinic, Women's College Hospital
Toronto, Canada

For many years, Dr. Stein's patients in and around Calgary have had the opportunity to attend a series of groups on managing the symptoms of ME/CFS, FM and MCS. She has now made a manual covering the important topics from this group. This will be of tremendous assistance to anyone considering setting up psychotherapeutic or support groups. It will also be of tremendous assistance to individuals wanting to work through the various issues that they face. We would like to thank Dr. Stein for her work.

Margaret Parlor, President, National ME/FM Action Network

The manual, *Let Your Light Shine Through, Strategies for Living With Myalgic Encephalomyelitis/ Chronic Fatigue Syndrome, Fibromyalgia and Multiple Chemical Sensitivity [1st edition],* is very practical for patients who need to address multiple contributors, step by step!

Lynn Marshall, MD, FAAEM, LMCFP, Environmental Health Clinic,
Women's College Hospital

About the Author

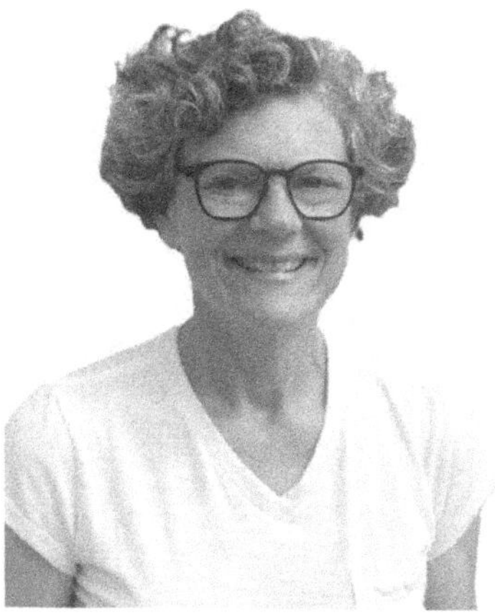

Dr. Eleanor Stein, MD, FRCP(C), is a Canadian psychiatrist whose career path shifted in 1989 when she developed myalgic encephalomyelitis/ chronic fatigue syndrome, fibromyalgia, environmental sensitivities, and chronic pain. For the next 25 years, she dedicated her practice to caring for people with complex chronic illness, including long COVID, since 2022.

After a significant improvement in her health in 2017, Dr. Stein became an even stronger advocate for science-based self-management strategies. Since retiring from clinical practice in 2023, she has dedicated her efforts to online education, empowering people around the world to take charge of their healing.

Her website, www.eleanorsteinmd.ca, offers a wealth of **free** resources and paid courses. This manual is the foundation for her self-management course, *Pathways to Improvement*. Due to the success of that course and her ever-growing knowledge, she developed two courses teaching neuroplasticity: *Healing Through Neuroplasticity and Rewiring Your Brain*. In 2024, she launched a subscription-based membership called *Live! with Dr. Stein*. This program features live sessions every other Thursday via Zoom, where Dr. Stein shares insights from her 35 years of medical practice, boosted by cutting-edge science and strategies that have the power to change your life. She answers participants' questions in every session. For people interested in meeting live with one of the most experienced physicians in the field of complex chronic diseases, visit www.eleanorsteinmd.ca/live.

About the Editor

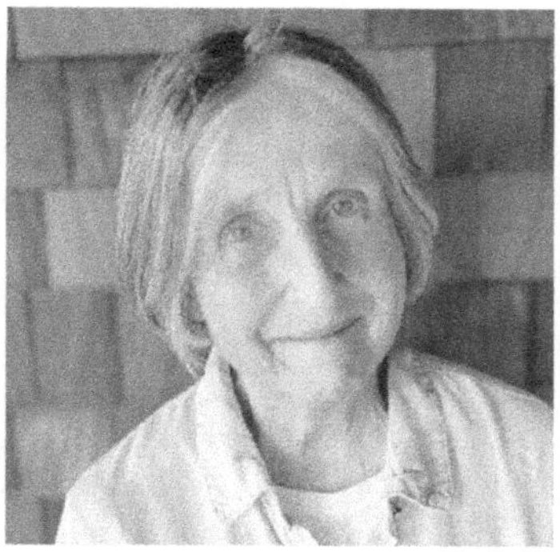

Maureen MacQuarrie edited this manual in 2012 and, at the time, marvelled at the amazing collection of resources it contained. Almost a decade and a half later, its contents are still relevant. Although still sidelined by ME/ CFS, Maureen has been helped by many of the strategies it contains, and she is delighted that the manual is being reprinted and will be accessible to more people. Maureen now calls Collingwood, Ontario, Canada, home.

Content

Cover Pages

Charts and Tools

Go to the link to download and print as many copies as you need: www.eleanorsteinmd.ca/tools

Introduction

Introduction

Welcome to this manual. The introduction will explain why I wrote the manual and how I hope it can be useful to patients with ME/CFS, FM, and MCS, as well as to health care professionals who want to learn more.

Manual Title

It was so hard to choose a title for this manual. I decided to open suggestions to the patient and advocate community, and was flooded with excellent suggestions. The themes of the entries fell into a few categories. Several had to do with surviving (e.g., "ME/CFS, FM and MCS Survival Guide," "Surviving and Thriving" with these conditions). Then there were several suggestions about taking charge, overcoming adversity, and creating health. These are all strong, attractive ideas.

And then there were the ideas about moving from the fog or darkness into the light. This theme became suddenly more compelling when I happened upon what would become the cover artwork for the first edition, a watercolor of Castle Mountain in a Banff, Alberta art store. Suzan de Laine, the artist of *Castle Mountain,* said in the short bio that accompanied her work that, being a former stained-glass artist, she strives to "let the light shine through" her pictures. And the picture had blue, purple and green as the dominant colors: the colors representing ME/CFS, FM and MCS, respectively. It seemed like such a gift.

With ME/CFS, FM and MCS, life can become very foggy and dark due to the severity of symptoms and the sheer lack of energy. Many people feel they have lost themselves or lost their way by the time they stumble into my office. When Suzan responded to my request to collaborate on the cover for the manual, the theme was set. We kept the theme of light in the second edition but simplified the cover to optimize for mobile scrolling online.

The manual title symbolizes that there is hope. Our inner light is always there, even on the "darkest" day. By the end of working through this manual, I hope you will be better connected with your own light and that it will be shining brighter for you and those around you. The title also suggests that the solutions or "light" we are searching for are within us and not outside. I can guide patients to certain treatments and attitudes which may help them, but to "feel better," you must find and utilize inner resources to forge your own path from illness to health. And yes...you have those resources.

Some of the additional submissions I received, including title suggestions, photos, and some poetry, are included at the start of each session (chapter). I think these additions add soul to the manual. We are, after all, more than our bodies. A big thank you to everyone who contributed, including those whose ideas weren't included.

Why Focus on Management Strategies Rather Than a Cure?

When asked, the patients I work with all tell me that they would like to "get better." By this, they mean "I want improved health, so that my life can return to what it was like before I became ill." The good news is that symptom management strategies, including those discussed in this manual, can make a profound and significant difference in quality of life.

Management strategies, including lifestyle changes, medications and nutritional supplementation, are all impacting the body downstream of the causes of ME/CFS, FM and MCS and are not generally curative. However, virtually all patients, and not only those with these conditions, can attain a better level of psychological and physical health through learning about their own bodies and making changes accordingly. In other words, despite all the complexities of and controversies surrounding these conditions, there is hope.

Scope of the Manual

This manual combines information with questions and exercises designed to get readers thinking about the factors that are contributing to their symptoms and what they can do to change them.

- In several sessions, I include lists of the medication strategies that I find most useful. To pursue these options, you will need to work with a medical doctor (MD) as medications must be prescribed by a qualified professional.
- In some of the sessions, I include information on tests commonly used in Environmental and Functional medicine, which are not publicly funded by the Canadian health care system.

This manual is not an exhaustive review of self-management strategies, medications, side effects, or testing. It is a summary of those strategies that I find the most useful in my practice with real patients (i.e., as opposed to research subjects). The people who come to see me have often been ill for some time and have complicated medical histories with symptoms that often can't be explained by conventional medicine. My patients may not be reflective of every patient with ME/CFS, FM and MCS. As you read, keep in mind that this manual reflects the world of ME/CFS, FM and MCS through the lens of my experience.

Each session covers one important topic experienced by most people with complex chronic diseases: diagnosis, sleep, activity, coping, diet, toxic exposures, pain and mental health. In my experience, most people with these conditions need to address many of the topic areas covered in this manual to improve their health. You may also suffer from symptoms not discussed in this manual. This does not mean these symptoms are less important, only that they are less common and do not need to be addressed in all patients.

The final session compiles a list of eight of the most commonly used and effective interventions in the fields of ME/CFS, FM and MCS. These common treatments require you to work with a qualified medical or naturopathic doctor. It is not advisable to embark on these tests or treatments alone.

The manual is written primarily for patients and contains enough medical references to assist practitioners who want to learn more.

Readers whose primary diagnosis is environmental sensitivity (ES), either sensitivity to chemicals or electromagnetic radiation, may be disappointed that references to these conditions occur less frequently than do references to ME/CFS or FM. Multiple chemical sensitivity (MCS) and electromagnetic hypersensitivity (EHS) are dealt with primarily in Session 6: Lowering the Toxic Load. In general, people with MCS and EHS will also benefit from the other recommendations, but for them, avoiding exposure and the recommendations in Session 6 are the most important.

The manual was developed from handouts I created for groups I ran in my medical practice since the early 2000s. If you do not live in Calgary or even in Alberta or Canada, you may not have access to some of the services mentioned. Alternatively, you may have access to some services that are not mentioned, and you may be wondering why they are left out. I have limited the recommendations to strategies that are available to my patients, as it is frustrating to read about things that one can't access. Please consider the recommendations as illustrations of what might be possible if sufficient, appropriate resources were available.

Children and Adolescents

The manual does not mention how to diagnose or support children and adolescents with ME/CFS, FM or MCS. ME/CFS and FM are well-documented in school-aged children and adolescents, though both conditions are far less common in youth than in adults. With a few exceptions, the symptoms of these conditions in children and adolescents are similar to those in adults. Experts suggest a shorter mandatory duration of symptoms before diagnosis can be made (e.g., three months instead of six for ME/CFS). A pediatric definition for ME/CFS has been published (Jason et al., 2006) based on the Canadian Case Definition. The American Pain Society has several publications that include the diagnosis and management of FM in children and adolescents, including their *2005 Clinical Practice Guidelines* (American Pain Society, 2005). I am not aware of any literature on the prevalence, diagnosis, or management of MCS or ES in children or adolescents.

I do not have experience working with pre-adolescents with these conditions, though I am aware both from the literature and from the experiences of other practitioners that they do exist. The charting tools discussed throughout the manual are often too onerous for children or adolescents to complete independently.

Around age 17 - 18, most teens begin to take a more autonomous interest and role in their own health care, and at that point, most are able to use the charting tools to benefit. For younger patients, the manual may be best used by parents who will then discuss certain aspects as appropriate with their child and the child's physician.

The *TEACH-ME* manual (https://www.mefmaction.com/index.php?option=com_content&view=article&id=288&Itemid=356), published by the National ME/FM Action Network and available on their website, is a guide for teachers of young people with ME/CFS and FM. It discusses the impact of ME/CFS and FM on education and suggests some strategies for accommodation that can assist affected students in completing and succeeding at their education.

Who Should Use This Manual?

This manual is not just for beginners (i.e., those new to these illnesses). People who have been ill for many years will benefit from using the manual as an update, a review, and a chance to re-evaluate their symptom patterns to see if they have changed. ME/CFS, FM and MCS are not static conditions.

Groups are very powerful. In a group, you can pool resources and ideas to let you know you are not alone. You could join my community to connect with others or find like-minded people online. If none of these options is available to you, I recommend working through the manual by yourself at the pace suggested (if you are able). Keep in mind that you are not alone. There are many others like you, and their experience has made this manual possible.

How to Use This Manual

The order of the sessions in this manual has evolved over the years I have facilitated groups. In my opinion, each session is essential. You must consider and manage each of these common symptom areas to progress towards better health. In general, you should deal with the worst symptoms first. For most people, these are sleep, fatigue (activity), and diet/gut.

However, if you are someone for whom stress or psychological symptoms are a priority, you may choose to start with these sessions first and work your way back. If you are not sure where to start, I suggest working through the manual in order. If you have a burning issue that cannot wait, then start there. In many cases, you may judge that you need help beyond the scope of self-management. In that case, please seek additional assistance from local practitioners.

Many people ask why pain is left until towards the end. This is because pain is very difficult to deal with directly. Only after other aspects of management are improved can you really make an impact on pain. If you start with Session 7 on pain, you are unlikely to be successful until you improve the management of other symptoms.

Each session ends with a section called "Preparing for Session (next)." This will explain which charts you need and how to record your health information in preparation for the next session.

You will follow along with a typical but fictional character, "Joan." From Joan's charting, you will be able to learn how to complete the self-observation charts and what to look for in your own data.

Before reading each new session, other than Sessions 1 and 9, it is strongly recommended that you spend two weeks getting to know and recording the aspect of your functioning that will be discussed in that session. You will learn much more by reading each session only after you have carefully observed your activities and symptoms for two weeks. In this way, you will follow along as if you were in a live group and gain some of the same benefits from new awareness.

In my experience, it is much better to chart your symptoms before you read the next session. This ensures that you are not being biased by what you read. Therefore, even though it is very tempting to read ahead and learn as much as possible as quickly as possible, I strongly advise against it.

If you follow the guidelines for using this manual, it will take you at least 16 weeks to work through. There may be some patients who are 100% sure that they have no problems in a certain area (e.g., diet and nutrition) and want to skip that session and not spend the two weeks prior to doing the charting. I advise against skipping chapters and their accompanying charting.

I encourage you to make as many copies of the tools and charts as you require for personal use. Please remember that all the material in this manual is copyrighted and cannot be copied for others without permission.

Charting

In Sessions 1 through 7, you will be introduced to a number of charts (or diaries) for the purpose of recording your activities and health symptoms and then transforming them into a visual format that will enable you to perceive your symptom profile more easily. Although charting is uniformly disliked, when the evaluations come in at the end of a group, it is generally noted as the most important tool for change!

When beginning charting, it is useful to establish a baseline score before you make any changes. As you read through the manual, you will get ideas for change. It is recommended that you continue with the self-observational charting after you decide on a change, to measure whether the changes you are making are beneficial.

A recurring theme of this manual is that not every recommendation will work for you. Some apparently innocuous interventions may make you feel worse in unexpected ways. There is no guaranteed or safe recommendation. Every intervention contains potential risks as well as benefits. You may need to try several strategies before finding ones that work for you. Consider this manual a buffet. Come back often and try many strategies to find the most effective for you.

In the manual, I will suggest ways in which you can modify the charts. You are encouraged to change them in any way that makes them more relevant and easier to use. They are for you, to enable you to discern patterns. Once you have chosen a particular chart, stick with it so that you can accurately compare your symptoms over time.

You may notice, as you use the charts, that your perception of your baseline self-ratings may. For example, many people overestimate their energy and functional capacity at the beginning. After charting for several weeks to months and noticing improvements, they wonder why their scores haven't changed. If this happens to you, you may find that you need to re-evaluate your starting point.

As you progress through the manual, there are occasions where you are asked to chart more than one aspect of your functioning at a time. The more effort you put into self-observation, the more you will glean about the connection between your various symptoms and between your activities and your symptoms. Many of you have limited energy and may feel overwhelmed charting more than one symptom at a time. Indeed, even charting one symptom can be very draining. In that case, do what you can. It is better to gather information slowly than to set too large a goal and experience a relapse as a result. As with everything else related to ME/CFS, FM and MCS, try to find a balance that works for you.

How to Use Your Completed Self-Observation Charts

At various times, as you work through this manual and certainly at the end after you have gathered information on each of the important symptom clusters, I suggest pulling out all your charts and lining them up on a large table (or on your computer, depending on how you have gathered your information). Start with the *Sleep Charts*. Study the graphs at the bottom and look for patterns. You especially want to notice what activities or events occurred in the day or days before changes in symptoms. For example, if you had an especially good or bad day, study what you did in the days before that day to generate ideas about what may have led to the good day.

If you are plotting two or more symptoms (e.g., pain and sleep), ask yourself the following questions:

- Are the lines parallel to each other?
- Are they a mirror image?
- Does one line change, and then the other similarly shifts a day or more later?
- Do the symptom lines seem entirely unrelated?

If one symptom seems to precede another, it may be that one problem is causing the other. In this case, in developing a management plan, you would choose the causative symptom to work on. For example, if you notice that after several nights of bad sleep, your pain increases, you may conclude that poor sleep is contributing to increased pain. In this case, you would focus on improving your sleep, hoping that the pain will lessen as a result.

If two symptoms are related to each other and change at the same time, start by working on the one that feels easiest to improve. For example, if pain and sleep vary like a mirror image (more pain and less sleep), you could address either symptom and, as you improve it, the other may also improve. High pain can interfere with sleep, and poor sleep increases pain.

Using the *Activity Log* and *Activity and Symptoms Chart* does not provide the advantage of visual graphs to show patterns. Instead, you must carefully read through the list of activities that seem most commonly associated with adverse effects. Those are the ones to address first since you will benefit the most if they can be changed. For example, if being around a certain person always leads to you feeling worse, you may decide to do an experiment and spend less time with that person. If a certain store gives you a headache, try avoiding it or if you must go in, wear a filter mask. If certain types of activity predictably worsen your pain or your sleep, try to figure out a different way to accomplish the same task.

Readers' Responsibilities

The reader remains responsible for researching all the suggestions in this manual and discussing them with a licensed health care professional to ensure suitability and safety.

- If I have learned anything over the past 11 years, it is that each patient is an individual and no recommendation works in every case. Did I already mention this? It cannot be repeated too often.
- Many people hold the false belief that pharmaceutical drugs are inherently harmful, whereas natural remedies are safe. This is simply not true. **Any intervention that has the power to heal also has the power to harm**.
- Read on at your own risk and find a health care provider who can assist you.

The fields of ME/CFS, FM and MCS are filled with controversies. There is a spectrum of views ranging from those who believe that these conditions are serious medical conditions requiring medical intervention to those who believe that they are not serious and/or are primarily psychological in origin.

For the record, I believe that ME/CFS, FM and MCS are serious medical conditions. Unfortunately, research is lagging far behind the needs of the community. The symptom management strategies in this manual do not address the underlying medical issues. However, we all make small lifestyle decisions every day that affect our quality of life. This manual may help you consider what you can do to improve your quality of life. As you do more reading on the various topics, you will find material with different perspectives. You will have to judge how the material applies to your situation.

Disclosures

- I do not benefit in any way from the recommendations contained in this manual and have no financial interest in any of the products or services recommended.
- Since 2010, I have been a medical advisor to the National ME/FM Action Network, a voluntary, unpaid position.
- I became interested in ME/CFS, FM and MCS because I contracted this constellation of conditions in 1989. It has taken me many years of reading, conferences, personal experimentation and working with patients to optimize my own health. It continues to be a daily struggle. (See Preface to the 2025 Edition below.)
- Some believe that this personal involvement is a benefit; that I can better understand the symptoms and challenges of the relentless struggle to function and enjoy life in the face of these conditions.
- Others believe that having an illness precludes scientific objectivity.
- Both views contain some elements of truth.

Acknowledgements

I wish to thank all the patients with ME/CFS, FM and MCS who have chosen to work with me over the past 11 years and have taught me many of the strategies discussed in this manual. A big thank you goes to Maureen MacQuarrie, who has painstakingly edited this manual. Maureen has spent many, many hours helping me revise each session to be clear, complete, and consistent. What you are reading is immeasurably better for her input.

Eleanor Stein, MD, FRCP(C)
Calgary, Canada
May 2012

Looking towards the day when every patient with ME/CFS, FM, and MCS in Canada receives prompt, respectful and effective health care and social support.

Preface to the 2025 Edition

Since writing this manual in 2011/2012, I have learned a huge amount about ME/CFS, FM, MCS (now expanded to environmental sensitivities or ES) and the other conditions commonly associated with these diagnoses, things like postural orthostatic tachycardia syndrome (POTS), mast cell activation syndrome (MCAS), small intestinal bacterial overgrowth (SIBO) and others.

I share a wealth of new material on my website (https://www.eleanorsteinmd.ca/) in the form of blogposts and short videos.

Despite being 13 years old, the information in this manual remains accurate, up to date, and useful, with a few exceptions. Self-management remains a keystone to healing, and the strategies discussed in this manual have been tried and tested. This 2nd edition is not a full rewrite. I omitted outdated sections and added new ones where significant advances have occurred.

In this second edition,

- the resource links have been checked and updated.
- outdated material has been deleted.
- some local references to Calgary, Canada, have been deleted, making the content relevant to global readers.
- new material has been added to reflect updates in science and consensus guidelines.
- a new bonus session has been added, featuring some of the exciting information I am learning, all evidence-based and packed with no-to-low-cost self-management strategies.

The number of people experiencing ME/CFS has significantly increased because of the COVID pandemic. Estimates of the risk of developing long COVID after an acute SARS-CoV-2 infection vary widely from about 4% – 36%. Over 400 million people have contracted COVID worldwide. This means that tens of millions now have long COVID, and many of them report symptoms indistinguishable from ME/CFS. Regardless of how you developed ME/CFS, the practical, accessible guidance offered in this manual is relevant and helpful for you.

Over the past 25 years, I have become an even stronger advocate of self-management using simple, accessible lifestyle strategies. Despite exciting, ongoing research, biomedical treatment has yet to make a dent in the symptom burden of those suffering from what is now called complex chronic disease (ME, CFS, FM, ES, long COVID and others).

Please don't wait; learn about your condition and try some of the strategies in this manual.

If I can leave you with one message, it is that there is hope. Since writing this manual, I have experienced a significant improvement in my own health due to some of the strategies I share in this manual. With holistic self-management, better health is the rule, not the exception.
https://www.eleanorsteinmd.ca/about-story

To read about my story or learn more about any of the topics in this manual, please go to my website https://www.eleanorsteinmd.ca/, where you can access both free curated resources and courses to guide you further.

Ellie Stein
Calgary, Canada
September 2025

Introduction References

American Pain Society. Guideline for the Management of Fibromyalgia Syndrome Pain in Adults and Children. [4], 1-107. 2005. Glenview, Illinois, American Pain Society. Ref Type: Report

Bested, A.C. & Logan, A.C. (2008). *Hope and Help for Chronic Fatigue Syndrome and Fibromyalgia,* 2nd edn, Cumberland House, Nashville, Tennessee.

Jason, L.A., Bell, D.S., Rowe, K., Van Hoof, E., Jordan, K., Lapp, C., Gurwitt, A., Teruhisa, M., Torres-Harding, S., & De Meirleir, K. (2006). A pediatric case definition for Myalgic Encephalomyelitis and Chronic Fatigue Syndrome. *Journal of Chronic Fatigue Syndrome,* 13, 1-53.

Session 1

Laying the Foundation

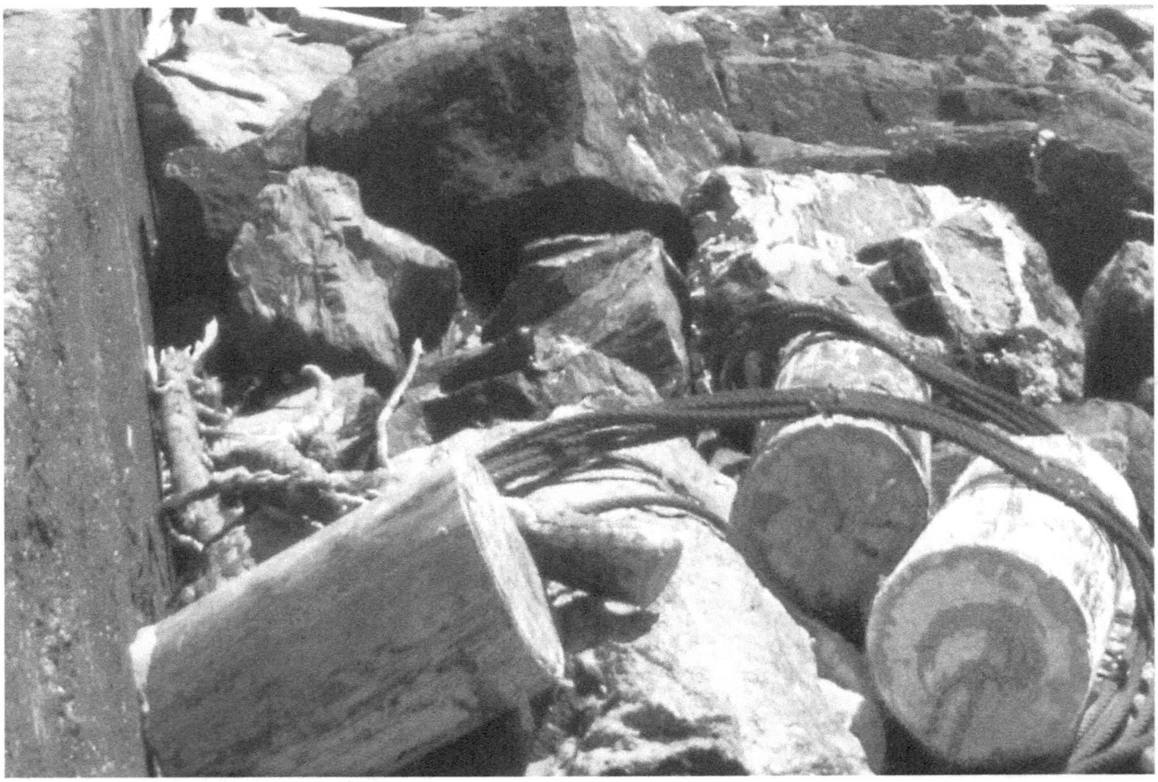

Diagnosis

It sneaks up on you. You feel terrible. One day you wake up and realize that you are living a nightmare.
It feels like your body parts are gripped by steel bands.
There is a jumble of symptoms, sharp, nasty and debilitating.
Pain and fatigue are your new life.
You seek a diagnosis and what you get is a stone wall.
Finally you find a doctor that listens and you take step one on the road to wellness.

The Road Well Traveled Part I

Session 1

Laying the Foundation

Objectives

- Understanding the benefits of self-management.
- Learning to set achievable goals.
- Getting to know your body, what makes you feel better and what makes you feel worse.
- Evaluating whether your illness experience fits the profile of any (or all) of ME/CFS, FM or MCS.

Introduction

Myalgic encephalomyelitis/chronic fatigue syndrome (ME/CFS), fibromyalgia (FM) and multiple chemical sensitivity (MCS) are clinical diagnoses. This means that there is no pathognomonic (100% proof) test for any of these conditions. The diagnoses are made by careful history taking, a physical exam, and laboratory investigations to rule out other possible causes of the symptoms and by assessing whether your profile matches the profiles commonly seen in these conditions. While the *core diagnostic symptoms* of these three disorders are different, the conditions do share overlapping symptoms and benefit from some of the same management strategies. Most readers will therefore appreciate the three conditions being considered together. Wherever possible, I identify which conditions are being specifically referred to.

The diagram on the next page was prepared using data obtained from Statistics Canada's 2014 *Canadian Community Health Survey* (CCHS). The Canadian Community Health Survey randomly sampled Canadians over the age of 12, asking them to indicate which of a list of chronic health conditions they had been diagnosed with. This list includes ME/CFS, FM, MCS, stroke, heart disease, cancer and others. You will see in this diagram that the results of the survey show that over 1,428,000 Canadians have been diagnosed with one or more of ME/CFS, FM and/or MCS. You are NOT alone. In my opinion, this survey probably underestimates the comorbidity among the three conditions. In other words, patients whom I see are more likely than not to have more than one of these conditions. Since the CCHS is a self-report survey, it may be that participants were unaware of other diagnoses.

Prevelance of Myalgic Encephalomyelitis/Chronic Fatigue Syndrome (ME/CFS) , Fibromyalgia (FM) and Multiple Chemical Sensitivities (MCS) in Canada (2014)

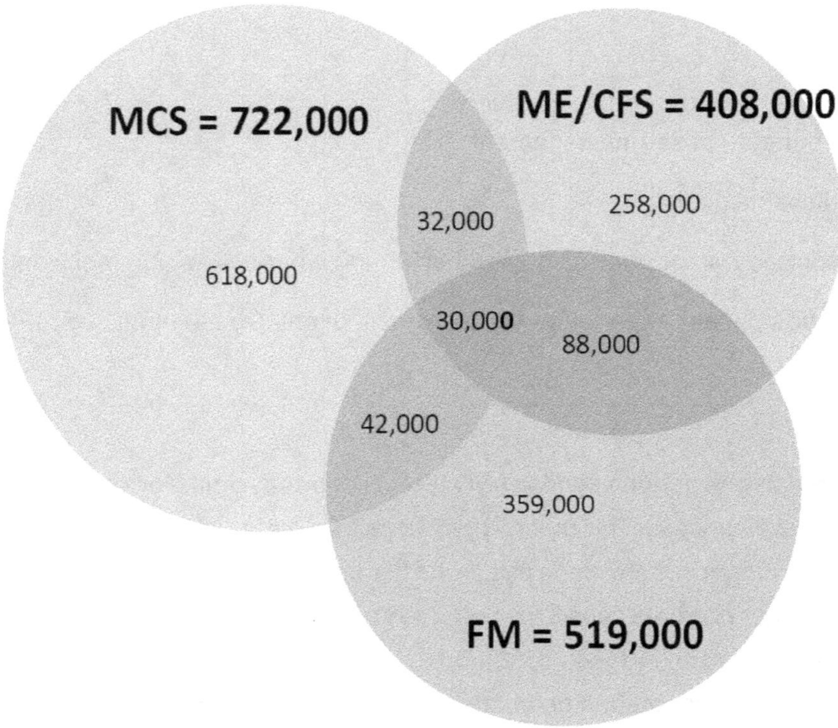

Total reporting one or more diagnosis: 1,428,000

Source: Statistics Canada Canadian Community Health Survey 2014, Public Use Microdata File
Compiled by the National ME/FM Action Network

These data are used with permission of the National ME/FM Action Network.

As mentioned in the Introduction, the number of people with ME/CFS has increased dramatically since the COVID pandemic and the transition of so many from acute to long COVID. One estimate is that approximately 3.3% of the Canadian adult population suffers from long COVID (Zakaria, Demers, Cheta, Aziz, & Abdullah, 2025). This translates into as many as 660,000 additional cases of ME/CFS in Canada.

Nomenclature (definitions)

It's always a bad sign when people can't agree on what to call a condition. Conditions that are well understood generally have a name that is descriptive of the condition, and those names are not generally contested. In this manual, I have chosen to use the terms myalgic encephalomyelitis/chronic fatigue syndrome (ME/CFS), fibromyalgia (FM) and multiple chemical sensitivity (MCS). I'll say more about the actual conditions in the "Do You Have ME/CFS, FM and/or MCS?" section on pages 1-10.

FM: The term fibromyalgia (FM) is fairly well accepted as a descriptor of the condition.

ME: Myalgic encephalomyelitis (ME) is a term that was coined in the 1950s to describe patients who had become ill in several epidemics, including one at the Royal Free Hospital in London (Acheson, 1959). The symptom profile of ME includes profound fatigue and muscle weakness.

CFS: Chronic Fatigue Syndrome (CFS) was described by the Centers for Disease Control criteria of 1988 (Holmes et al., 1988) in response to an illness outbreak at Lake Tahoe. The Holmes definition was revised in 1994 by Fukuda et al (Fukuda et al., 1994).

ME/CFS: ME/CFS is an umbrella term that includes patients with ME and those with CFS. The *Canadian Consensus Criteria* (Carruthers et al., 2003) chose to combine these conditions and call them ME/CFS. There were many reasons for this decision, including dissatisfaction with the name CFS. One criticism is that although a number of symptoms are necessary for the diagnosis of ME/CFS, the name CFS focuses only on fatigue. Another is that the term CFS doesn't communicate the seriousness of the condition.

Systemic Exertion Intolerance Disease (SEID): The Institute of Medicine (IOM, now called the National Academy of Medicine) was tasked by the National Institutes of Health in the United States to exhaustively review the medical literature for the purpose of making recommendations on how best to define and diagnose ME/CFS (Institute of Medicine, 2015). They used the Canadian Consensus Criteria as a starting point.

In their comprehensive 2015 report, the IOM proposed a new definition to encourage front-line practitioners to make the diagnosis. The SEID criteria specify that symptoms must be present at least half the time and with at least moderate intensity. In my experience, most patients have symptoms 100% of the time.

Since its publication in 2015, the IOM/NAC criteria have gained widespread acceptance, but the name SEID has not stuck. Most people refer to these criteria as the *IOM/NAM ME/CFS criteria*.

In this manual, I use the term ME/CFS in the way defined in the 2003 Canadian Consensus Criteria.

MCS: I use the term multiple chemical sensitivity (MCS) to refer to illness triggered by small amounts of chemicals. In this manual, I have used the term MCS as per the 1999 international definition, as described at the end of this session, and the condition is discussed in detail in Session 6. MCS is only one form of environmental illness. In this manual, I often use the umbrella term *environmental illness* or *environmental sensitivity* (ES).

Environmental Toxicity: Environmental toxicity is another problematic environmental health concern. Environmental toxicity includes all health conditions that are caused by or worsened by exposure to toxins such as petrochemicals, mercury, dioxins, hydrofluorocarbons, and others, either man-made or released due to human activity. Environmental toxicity is an increasingly serious and ubiquitous problem. Environmental toxicity, while important, is not discussed in this manual because many conditions caused by environmental toxicity (e.g., asthma, heart disease, and cancer) are not in the family of or related to ME/CFS, FM and MCS. Diagnosis and treatment of environmental toxicity are taught in the field of environmental medicine. You can refer to the American Academy of Environmental Medicine http://www.aaemonline.org/ or the International Society of Environmentally Acquired Illness https://iseai.org/ for more information.

EHS: Electromagnetic Hypersensitivity (EHS) is included in Session 6 as an emerging illness. It is possible that people with ME/CFS, FM and MCS may also be vulnerable to developing EHS, although it is too early to know since research on this condition is in its infancy.

Illness Severity

Researching ME/CFS, FM and MCS is difficult because of the variable presentation in different people and the variable presentation in one person from day to day. A small number of patients with ME/CFS are mildly affected and can manage household chores, do errands, see friends and work outside the home (though never all on the same day). Since the definition of ME/CFS requires physical and mental fatigue that substantially reduces activity level (in some definitions by 50%), very few patients can work.

A subgroup of people with ME/CFS are so ill as to be bedbound or housebound and dependent upon others for daily care. This group is referred to as the 25% group, as their energy and function are less than 25% of what it was when they were healthy. For more information relevant to the most severely ill, go to the UK-based 25% ME group. https://25megroup.org/

The spectrum of illness severity in FM is likewise vast. Some patients have a bothersome daily achiness and must limit exercise, but can otherwise pass for normal. Others have such severe pain that they are severely limited both by the pain and the impact of the pain on energy, sleep and mood.

Some people with MCS are able to go out in public and attend social functions if they take certain precautions, such as ensuring that others present don't wear scented products. Others with MCS are essentially housebound because they have such severe reactions to any chemical they are exposed to, and these exposures are unavoidable.

Similarly, patients with EHS can be mildly affected and function normally as long as they limit cell phone and computer time. Others live without major appliances, with the power turned off in their homes and undertake expensive shielding to limit exposures from their neighbours.

Daily Symptom Variability

One of the most difficult aspects of managing and living with ME/CFS, FM and MCS is the unpredictability of daily symptom patterns. Symptoms in these conditions can change quickly in reaction to what most people would consider small stressors (e.g., preparing lunch, taking a shower, or exposure to a toner cartridge or a cell phone). Whereas most medical conditions, such as heart disease or arthritis, progress slowly and are quite predictable from day to day, symptoms in ME/CFS, FM and MCS can change on a dime. This means that planning ahead is difficult. Patients often have to cancel plans or back out of commitments at the last minute because of a sudden change in health, even after months of stability.

Patients often report feeling more vulnerable than others. They feel vulnerable to infection, temperature, barometric pressure, stress, activities and more. And they report that recovering from setbacks takes longer than expected (even after years of experience). The ease of precipitating a relapse and the difficulty of the struggle to recover can be very disheartening.

Self-management helps. Patients who are more aware of their relapse triggers can attempt to avoid or moderate them. By having more stable days due to optimal self-management, resilience to unexpected stressors increases.

Why Practice Self-Management?

Self-management refers to strategies that you can implement yourself. This process starts with careful and dispassionate self-observation of your symptoms. Since it is difficult for most people (even healthy ones) to remember many observations over time, it is best to make written notes about daily health patterns. This is referred to in this manual as *charting*.

In the Introduction, I provided some ideas about how to begin charting and also what to look for once the charts are completed. In doing this, you begin to notice what makes you feel better or worse. Virtually every patient who devotes time to charting learns valuable information about themselves.

Using this information, you can formulate hypotheses (hunches) about things that might help your particular symptoms. Then you can try interventions and monitor the results. Charting is part of routine treatment in most chronic health conditions, specifically chronic pain and chronic sleep disorders. Why? Because it works.

Self-management has proven helpful in virtually every biomedical condition in which its use has been studied, including arthritis (most studied), heart disease, multiple sclerosis, and cancer. Self-management allows individuals to take their lives into their own hands; it increases empowerment, and people feel better, too!

Self-management alone may not cure anyone of ME/CFS, FM or MCS. However, to paraphrase a quote from the veteran ME/CFS doctor, Dr. Charles Lapp, "there is no drug that can surpass the impact of thoughtful self-management." If one does not learn to notice the messages the body is sending and respond accordingly, one will not recover. If one optimizes self-management, improvement is possible. For most patients, self-management is necessary but not sufficient for recovery of health and function.

In a study of a psychoeducational group therapy for fibromyalgia, people attending the group (as compared to people getting usual medical care) reported less physical impairment, pain, general fatigue, stiffness, anxiety, and depression (Luciano et al., 2011). In medical research, a statistic called *number needed to treat* (NNT) is used to describe how powerful an intervention is. For many drugs (e.g., antidepressants, drugs to lower cholesterol and prevent heart disease, etc.), it is required to treat between 5 and 11 people to ensure statistically that one will get better. Yes, you read correctly. For the most effective medical treatments, between 5 and 11 patients need to be treated for one patient to improve over and above the placebo rate. In the psychoeducational group treatment of FM mentioned above, the number needed to treat was 3. This suggests that self-management can be a powerful intervention.

Getting to Know Your Body

Self-observation is essential since no one is better suited than you to figure out what is going on in your body. By charting daily and comparing your scores before and after you try something new, you can assess whether it worked or not. If you are not certain, run the experiment again—that is, stop the intervention, redo the baseline charting, and then retry the intervention. This is called an N of 1 trial (a study in which you are the only subject). If you again fail to be certain of a difference, then this intervention may not be effective for you. Move on to a new idea.

Often in group, patients ask me whether or not they should try a particular treatment. My answer is usually this, "If you are willing to undertake the health and financial risks involved, you should try it and notice whether it works or not." There is no intervention, apart from pacing, that consistently works for every patient. Therefore, a good deal of trial and error is required.

Goal Setting

Setting concrete, achievable goals to work on aids progress and maintains hope.

- If you set goals that are not measurable, you won't be able to assess whether your interventions have worked or not.
- If you set goals that are too difficult to achieve, you are likely to fail and become disillusioned.
- **ME/CFS, FM and MCS are so complicated and overwhelming that many people just give up and think nothing they can do will help. This is incorrect. Virtually every patient I have ever worked with has made some improvement.** Some, of course, make more progress than others depending on their circumstances and the severity and nature of their condition.

Goal setting is integral to the work of Dr. Kate Lorig and colleagues at Stanford School of Medicine. The textbook used in the Stanford Chronic Disease Self-Management Program is called *Living a Healthy Life with Chronic Conditions* (Lorig et al., 2007). The program described in Lorig's book has been shown to improve outcomes in many chronic conditions, including arthritis, heart disease, and diabetes.

In other words, in these conditions, there is strong evidence that self-management makes a difference. This book is now widely available at major booksellers and is an excellent complement to this manual. The book has a very useful section on goal setting called *Becoming an Active Self-Manager*. The specific suggestions recommended by Lorig and colleagues for goal setting are

1. Decide what you want to accomplish.
2. Look for an alternative way to accomplish it if your condition interferes.
3. Make a series of concrete short-term *action* plans.
4. Carry out your action plan(s) one at a time.
5. Assess the results.
6. Make changes as needed.
7. Reward yourself for achievements.

The most common error people make is setting goals that are too big to accomplish in the short term (e.g., losing 50 lbs.). This type of goal is only achievable if one breaks it into small steps and has a concrete action plan to achieve each step. Examples would be "don't eat after 8 pm tonight" or "walk for 10 minutes three times this week."

Set a goal that you are over 80% certain you can achieve. If your confidence is less than 80%, choose another goal that is more achievable. It is better to slowly achieve small successes than to set a large goal and fail. Success reinforces motivation, and motivation is a key to change.

The following quote, attributed to Mark Twain, summarizes goal setting nicely: "The secret of getting ahead is getting started. The secret of getting started is breaking your complex, overwhelming tasks into small, manageable tasks, and then starting on the first one."

Do You Have ME/CFS, FM and/or MCS?

The disease definitions included at the end of this session will help you and your health care professional clarify whether you fit one or more of the profiles for ME/CFS, FM or MCS. Since there is no gold standard test for any of these conditions, the diagnosis can only be made by a careful review of your history (ruling out other conditions which could be causing your symptoms), and by being intimately familiar with the most commonly used criteria. Read over the definitions and see if you think you fit the overall description.

If you need more information than provided here about ME/CFS, I recommend the National ME/FM Action Network website www.mefmaction.com. Here you will find the full report and the overview of *The Canadian Consensus Criteria (CCC)* also known as the *Myalgic Encephalomyelitis / Chronic Fatigue Syndrome: Clinical Working Case Definition, Diagnostic and Treatment Protocols.* These documents summarize the natural history of these two conditions and the mandatory symptoms for diagnosis. They also include valuable information about treatment and disability issues.

For more information on MCS, I recommend the following two Canadian summaries: *The Medical Perspective on Environmental Sensitivities,* written by Meg Sears for the Canadian Human Rights Commission (Sears, 2007) and *Environmental Sensitivities-Multiple Chemical Sensitivity Status Report,* written by the physicians of the Ontario Environmental Health Clinic at Women's College Hospital in Toronto (Marshall et al., 2011).

If, after reading these definitions, you and your health care professional believe that any or all ME/CFS, FM or MCS accurately describes your health problems, then the information in this manual may be of benefit to you. If, after reading the definitions, you find significant differences between your health profile and those in the definitions, you should talk to your physician about finding an alternative explanation for your symptoms.

You will notice that there is more than one disease definition for ME/CFS and FM. This is because doctors and researchers don't yet agree 100% on the key symptoms that comprise each condition. As I noted in the section on nomenclature, as we learn more, new definitions are introduced. Each has pros and cons.

I classify every patient using both the Fukuda and Canadian definitions for ME/CFS. Most patients meet both criteria, but some meet only one and not the other. The Canadian definition is more specific and runs less risk of misdiagnosis (Jason et al., 2004). Since the first edition of this manual was published, the Canadian definition has supplanted the Fukuda in informed research.

For FM, there is no definition that is both specific (accurate) and widely accepted. For that reason, I use both the 1990 and 2010 American College of Rheumatology definitions for diagnosis. Session 6 deals with MCS. More about the definition of MCS and useful techniques for dealing with chemical and other environmental sensitivities can be found there.

Accessing Tests Not Covered by or Offered Through Provincial Health Care

Throughout this manual, I refer to some laboratory tests that many patients find useful to help guide their health decisions. However, most of these tests are not available in Canada. The tests that fall into this category generally provide information about nutrition and function rather than about the specific illness. You may find that your family physician is either unfamiliar with these tests or skeptical that the tests are valid and useful. Reputable laboratories require a requisition from a health care provider. This is because a knowledgeable health care professional, usually an MD or ND, is required to interpret the results. While this is not an exhaustive list, some physicians who are experienced with these tests are listed on the websites of environmental or functional medicine organizations.

Remember that no test is 100% accurate and that the test result may not show any problem (i.e., not explain why you are ill). Therefore, if considering a fee-for-service test, ask yourself how you will feel if the test result is negative or if it doesn't help you with your health decisions. Will you still feel it was worth the money spent? Never spend money on testing that you need for other things, such as rent and food and never spend money on testing that you can't afford to lose. Once you find a practitioner, be sure to inquire about the accuracy of the test and the relevance of the findings for your situation. Will the test result change your management plan?

Meet Joan

As a tool to help explain how to do the self-observational charting and how to interpret your information, we will follow along with a fictional patient, Joan. Joan has been diagnosed with fibromyalgia.

Joan is a 55-year-old woman who became ill several years ago after a skiing injury. She is 5'4" and currently weighs 160 pounds. After a few surgeries on her right ankle, she was left with chronic pain in the ankle, which later spread to become generalized pain and aching. She never recovered the energy and vitality she had prior to the accident. Slowly over the next couple of years, Joan developed other symptoms including decreased stamina, cognitive problems, muscle twitches, periodic abdominal cramps and diarrhea. She has problems with temperature regulation, and this interferes with her sleep. Because she is a "light sleeper," Joan is easily disrupted by noise.

Joan became unable to work a year after her accident. After two stressful years of advocating with her long-term disability provider through work, she was granted disability with the proviso that she also apply to the Canada Pension Plan. (CPP is the first payer. This means that private insurers will pay less if you are also receiving payments from CPP.) Obtaining approval from the CPP took an additional year. When this approval came through, the back pay all went to the private disability carrier.

It was a lot of work and stress, but Joan was lucky to have had a sympathetic human resources department at work helping her through the hurdles. Joan was successfully able to argue (both with her disability provider and with CPP) that, despite a lack of objective test results proving her condition, she was, nonetheless, unable to work enough hours to support herself above the poverty line. Even so, the process left her drained for a year or so.

Now, despite her ill health, Joan is attempting to work as a part-time bookkeeper to supplement her disability income. As you will see from the charting, Joan currently works two half days per week. This is within the annual income limit allowed by CPP.

Joan was dating at the time of her accident. After years of not being able to join her boyfriend for skiing and other outdoor activities, they split up. She now lives alone with her dog and has the responsibility of helping her aging parents negotiate health care and assisted living.

Joan's social life has suffered due to her decreased energy. She is now often unable to participate in previously enjoyed activities. She notices that she often feels ill after an evening out with friends and has cut back as a result. Because of her ankle pain and decreased ankle mobility, Joan has been unsuccessful in the exercise programs she has attempted. As a result, she is quite deconditioned and has gained 30 pounds since the accident.

Joan is lucky to have a family physician she likes. Joan's family physician attended a lecture on fibromyalgia and prescribed amitriptyline. Amitriptyline has helped with the pain and sleep, though her sleep is still unrefreshing. Joan's physician doesn't know what else to suggest next. Joan has been looking for information about what else she could do and stumbled across this manual. (Lucky Joan!) There are no specialized resources in Joan's locale, so Joan has been reading through it on her own and doing the charting exercises in each session. As you read the manual, you will learn alongside Joan as she learns about her symptoms.

Please remember, as you go through this manual, that every patient is an individual. The ideas that have helped Joan may also be helpful for many others, but they may not be true for you. Use your own judgment and discuss any interventions you plan to try with your health care professional before you try them.

Preparing for Session 2

Before reading Session 2, take two weeks to record your sleep patterns.

You will need the following:

- Adapted Karnofsky Energy Rating Scale
- Sleep Chart

All the charting tools will be found in the Charts and Tools section at the end of the manual. To access a downloadable, printable file, go to www.eleanorsteinmd.ca/tools. You may make as many copies as you wish. Most people find completing the charts on paper easiest. Please note that the Sleep Chart asks you to record energy and pain, as well as sleep data.

A Note on the Adapted Karnofsky Energy Rating Scale

The *Karnofsky Rating Scale* was initially developed by Dr. Karnofsky, a cancer researcher, in 1948 (Karnofsky et al., 1948). He developed the scale to measure the health status (general well-being and activities of daily living) of cancer patients being treated with nitrogen mustards. This scale, in its original form, is used in some research to determine eligibility for inclusion in studies.

For ME/CFS research, participants are usually required to have a daily energy rating of 70% or below to be considered ill enough to be in a study. While useful for this purpose, most people with ME/CFS fall into the range between 50% and 70% on the original Karnofsky scale, meaning they are able to care for themselves but are unable to carry out normal activities or to work.

The Karnofsky scale has been adapted for use in ME/CFS so that the range of scores for the average patient is larger. This makes it easier to notice changes over time and to understand the impact of interventions. The first adaptation of the Karnofsky was made by Dr. David Bell, well known for his ongoing care of hundreds of young people who developed ME/CFS in an epidemic in Lyndonville, New York. He published his adaptation in a 1995 guide for physicians, one of the earliest publications in the field (Bell, 1995). Since the fatigue in ME/CFS is both mental and physical, Dr. Bell added descriptors to describe both mental and physical fatigue. Instead of falling into the narrow 60% - 70% range, most patients with ME/CFS fall into a range of 30% - 80% on the version of the Karnofsky scale adapted by Bell.

While a great step forward, I have found that even this adaptation is not a perfect instrument either. Some people have excellent mental stamina but very poor physical stamina, and vice versa. These patients have difficulty using this scale.

The version used in this manual is based on Dr. Bell's adaptation, with a few additional changes by me. I have added some descriptors to the Bell adapted scale to try to clarify what level of energy a person needs to be able to work part-time and full-time. Although developed for ME/CFS, I have found that this adapted energy rating scale is also of use for FM and MCS patients.

The Karnofsky Scale has also been adapted by Drs. Alison Bested and Lynn Marshall, two Toronto physicians who have made a huge contribution to the field. Their adaptation, renamed the *Functional Capacity Scale* is also a good scale and is widely used. I have included a copy of this in the Charts and Tools section in case you want to use it. The Functional Capacity Scale is on page 2 of the Activity Log (PDF).

Your choice of which scale to use is not as important as the consistent use of the same scale over time, so that you can assess if you are getting better or worse. I recommend selecting one of the existing scales or, if you feel none of them meet your needs, making one of your own. Once you choose a scale, stick with it and use it to observe your body more objectively.

The Sleep Chart

There are many sleep charts available. Most sleep and pain clinics have devised their own versions to meet the needs of their patients. The version used in this manual is adapted from the *Sleep Sheet* of Dr. Beverly Tompkins. She is a Calgary family physician who is a pioneer in the field of ME/CFS, FM and MCS. I moved to Calgary to work with her in 1998 and again in 2001. I have adapted her Sleep Sheet slightly, but of course, some people prefer the original version. The original is not available except from Dr. Tompkins.

Many of my patients have made their own charts to specifically note the variables that are of most interest to them. Such variables include mood, various types of pain, gastrointestinal symptoms, blood pressure, and heart rate. I'll be discussing these variables throughout this manual. Again, once you have chosen a chart, stick with it so that you can accurately compare your symptoms over time.

Joan's Sleep Chart

Joan, our fictional patient, has kept records for two weeks. A copy of her charting is shown on pages 1-15. You will note that Joan missed one day of charting when her father had an episode of chest pain and she accompanied her parents to the hospital. They had to wait several hours before he was seen, and she was exhausted when she got home.

As I noted in the Introduction, when beginning to chart, it is useful to establish a baseline score BEFORE you make any changes. To determine her baseline, Joan kept her bedtime medications the same every day and didn't make any changes to her nutritional supplements.

Carefully read the "Use of the Sleep Chart" explanation (p. 2 of the Sleep Chart). Then, using Joan's Sleep Chart as an example, record your own energy, pain, and sleep for the next 2 weeks. After converting the pain to a percentage, plot the results on the graph. Be gentle with yourself if you, like Joan, miss some time due to "life." Better to chart most days than not at all. We'll discuss Joan's Sleep Chart in Session 2.

Name Joan Smith **Date** Dec 12/11 **to** Dec 25/11
Meds: amitryptylline 20 mg
Supps: multi min / multi vit

Date	% Energy	Pain	Activities/other factors	HS Meds	Initiate mins	Depth	Aware	wake #/min	deep/ light	Refresh -ment
D12	60	4	work 4 hrs	Ami	45	3	S, T	2/45	4/3	P
13	55	5	doctor's appt	"	30	3	S, T	1/30	5/4	F
14	55	4	dinner out	"	90	2	S, T	4/60	3/4	P
15	45	6	work 4 hrs	"	60	3	S, T	2/30	4/4	P
16	45	6	rest day :)	"	45	3	S, T	2/30	5/4	P
17	55	5	errands		30	4	P, S	3/50	4/3	P
18	50	5	church, rest		60	3	P, S	2/40	3/3	P
19	55	4	work 4 hrs		50	3	P, T	2/45	3/4	P
20	50	4	took dog to vet STRESS!		80	3	—	1/20	5/3	P
21	50	4	walk with friends		60	3	P, T	2/50	7	P
22	55	6	work 4 hrs		45	4	S, T	1/30	4/4	P
23	60	5	father health crisis		80	3	S	3/60	3/3	P
24	—	—	too busy with father to		chart					
25	50	5	exhausted - rest day		60	3	S	2/50	5/3	P

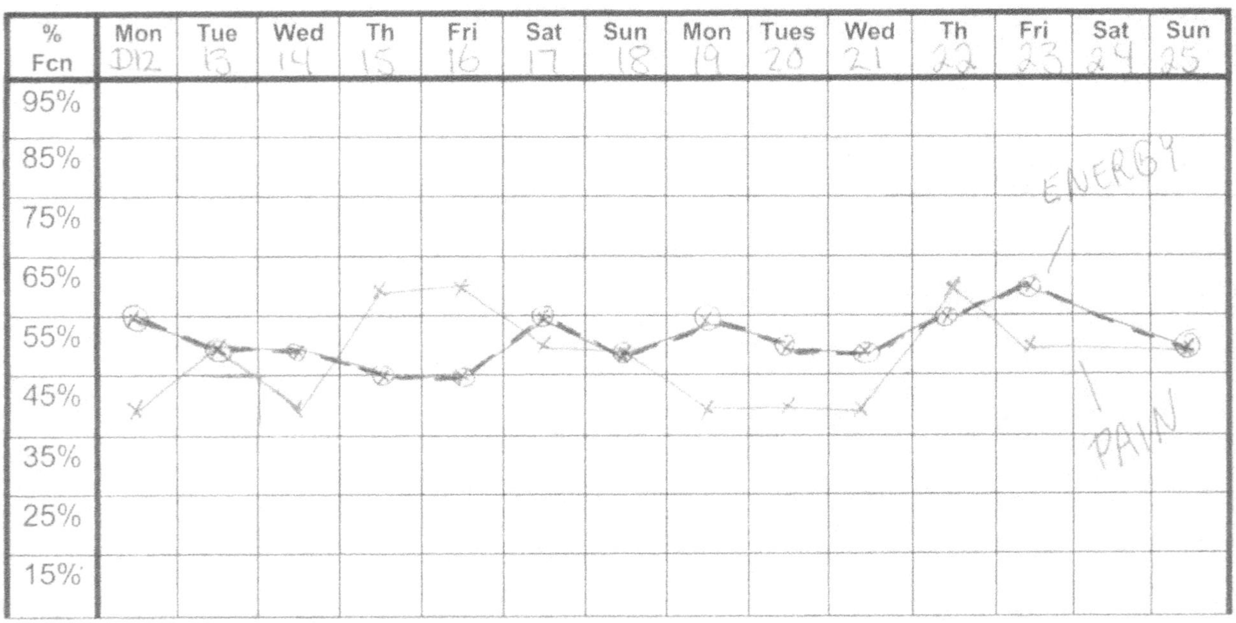

Adapted from the "sleep sheet" of Dr. Beverley Tompkins, Burke Institute, Calgary

Disease Definitions

1994 Centers for Disease Control Criteria for CFS

(Fukuda et al., 1994)

1. Unexplained, persistent fatigue (for at least 6 months) not improved substantially by rest and resulting in a substantially lower level of functioning than before the illness.

2. Four or more of the following for at least 6 months:

   - ☐ fatigue after mental or physical exertion that lasts more than 24 hours and is in excess of what would be expected when healthy
   - ☐ muscle pain
   - ☐ multi-joint pain without redness or swelling
   - ☐ problems with concentration, memory and/or mood
   - ☐ unrefreshing sleep
   - ☐ swollen or enlarged lymph nodes (glands)
   - ☐ sore throat
   - ☐ new or different headache

3. Although not included in the CDC criteria, most CFS patients also experience some of the following symptoms: abdominal pain, alcohol intolerance, bloating, chest pain, chronic cough, diarrhea, dizziness, dry eyes or mouth, earaches, irregular heartbeat, jaw pain, morning stiffness, nausea, night sweats, psychological problems (depression, irritability, anxiety, panic attacks), shortness of breath, skin sensations, and weight loss.

4. Other conditions that may cause fatigue must be ruled out or treated. These include hypothyroidism, sleep apnea and narcolepsy, depression, chronic mononucleosis, malnutrition/eating disorders, cancer, autoimmune disease, hormonal disorders, infections, alcohol or substance abuse, and reactions to prescribed medications.

2003 Canadian Consensus Definition of ME/CFS

(Carruthers et al., 2003)

1. Post-exertional Malaise and Fatigue

There is a loss of physical and mental stamina, rapid muscular and cognitive fatigability, post-exertional fatigue, malaise and/or pain, and a tendency for other symptoms to worsen. There is a pathologically slow recovery period (i.e., it takes more than 24 hours to recover). Symptoms are usually exacerbated by stress of any kind.

2. Fatigue

Patient must have a marked degree of new onset, unexplained, persistent or recurrent physical and mental fatigue that substantially reduces activity level.

3. Sleep Dysfunction

There is unrefreshed sleep or sleep quality and rhythm disturbance.

4. Pain

There is a significant degree of arthralgia and/or myalgia without clinical evidence of inflammatory responses of joint swelling or redness. The pain can be experienced in the muscles, joints, or neck and is often migratory in nature. Often, there are significant headaches of a new type, pattern, or severity.

5. Neurological/Cognitive Manifestations

Two or more of the following difficulties should be present: confusion, impairment of concentration and short-term memory consolidation, difficulty with information processing, categorizing and word retrieval, intermittent dyslexia, perceptual and sensory disturbances, disorientation, and ataxia. The patient may experience the *overload phenomena*—informational, cognitive and sensory, and/or emotional overload, which may lead to *crash* periods and/or anxiety.

6. At Least ONE Symptom Out of TWO of the Following Categories

a) *Autonomic Manifestations*

Orthostatic intolerance such as neurally mediated hypotension (NMH), postural orthostatic tachycardia syndrome (POTS), delayed postural hypotension, vertigo, lightheadedness, extreme pallor, intestinal or bladder disturbances with or without irritable bowel syndrome (IBS) or bladder dysfunction, cardiac arrhythmia, vasomotor instability, and respiratory irregularities.

b) *Neuro-endocrine Manifestations*

Loss of thermostatic stability, heat/cold intolerance, anorexia or abnormal appetite, marked weight change, hypoglycemia, loss of adaptability and tolerance for stress, worsening of symptoms with stress, slow recovery and emotional lability.

c) *Immune Manifestations*

Tender lymph nodes, sore throat, flu-like symptoms, general malaise, development of new allergies or changes in status of old ones and hypersensitivity to medications and/or chemicals.

7. The illness persists for at least six (6) months. It usually has a distinct onset, although it may be gradual. Preliminary diagnosis may be possible earlier. *Three months is appropriate for children.* To be included, the symptoms must have begun or have been significantly altered after the onset of the illness. It is unlikely that a patient will suffer from all symptoms in Criteria 4 and 5. The manifestations fluctuate and may change over time. Symptoms can exacerbate with stress, resulting in a slow rate of recovery. Children may experience numerous symptoms of similar severity, but their hierarchy of symptom severity tends to vary from day to day.

2015 National Academies of Medicine Diagnostic Criteria for ME/CFS (SEID)

(Institute of Medicine, 2015)

Diagnosis of ME/CFS requires the following three criteria to be met:

☐ **1. Substantial reduction or impairment in pre-illness levels of occupational, education, social, or personal activities that**

- persists for more than 6 months
- is accompanied by fatigue which is
  - often profound,
  - is of new or definite onset (not lifelong),
  - is not the result of ongoing excessive exertion,
  - is not substantially alleviated by rest.

☐ **2. Post-exertional malaise** at least half of the time with moderate, substantial, or severe intensity.

☐ **3. Unrefreshing sleep** at least half of the time with moderate, substantial, or severe intensity.

At least one of the following is also required:

☐ **Cognitive impairment** at least half of the time with moderate, substantial or severe intensity.

OR

☐ **Orthostatic intolerance**

For more information, https://nap.nationalacademies.org/resource/19012/MECFScliniciansguide.pdf

1990 American College of Rheumatology Definition of Fibromyalgia

(Wolfe et al., 1990)

The presence of pain, both above and below the waist, and on both sides of the body. This differentiates fibromyalgia from pain due to arthritis or injuries.

Duration of pain of at least 3 months to ensure it is not a transitory problem.

Pain at 11 or more of 18 designated tender point sites on physical exam.

Other conditions that may cause global muscular pain should be ruled out or treated. However, the presence of other disorders does not rule out the possibility of fibromyalgia.

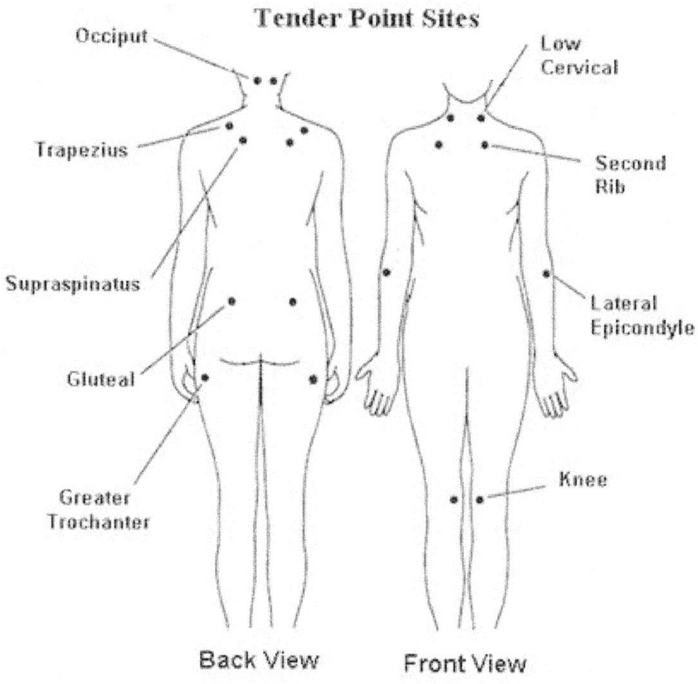

Fibromyalgia tender points diagram. U.S. Social Security Administration (2012). https://www.ssa.gov/OP_Home/rulings/di/01/SSR2012-02-di-01.html. Public domain.

2016 Diagnostic Criteria for Fibromyalgia

(Wolfe et al., 2016)

Widespread Pain Index (WPI)

One point for pain at each location In the last week.

REGION 1

Jaw
- ☐ Left

Shoulder girdle
- ☐ Left

Upper arm
- ☐ Left

Lower arm
- ☐ Left

REGION 2

Jaw
- ☐ Right

Shoulder girdle
- ☐ Right

Upper arm
- ☐ Right

Lower arm
- ☐ Right

REGION 3

Hip
- ☐ Left

Upper leg
- ☐ Left

Lower leg
- ☐ Left

REGION 4

Hip
- ☐ Right

Upper leg
- ☐ Right

Lower leg
- ☐ Right

REGION 5

- ☐ **Neck**
- ☐ **Upper back**
- ☐ **Chest**
- ☐ **Lower back**
- ☐ **Abdomen**

Widespread Pain Index (WPI) Total ____ /19

Symptom Severity Score (SSS)

Using the scale below, rate the severity of the symptoms in the last week.

____ **Fatigue**

____ **Unrefreshed sleep**

____ **Cognitive symptoms**

0	1	2	3
No symptoms	Slight/mild/ intermittent	Moderate/ often present	Severe/ pervasive/ continuous

Have the following been bothersome in the last month? (one point for each)

☐ **Headache** ☐ **Abdominal Pain** ☐ **Depression**

Symptom Severity Score (SSS) Total ____ /12

Fibromyalgia Severity Score = WPI + SSS = ____ **/31**

Diagnosis of fibromyalgia requires 3 conditions to be met:

1. **WPI ≥ 7 plus SSS ≥ 5 OR WPI ≥ 4 plus SSS ≥ 9.**
2. **Generalized pain i.e. pain in at least 4 of 5 regions (excluding jaw, chest, abdomen).**
3. **Symptoms present for at least 3 months.**

Dr. Eleanor Stein, MD FRCP(C)

International Consensus Definition for Multiple Chemical Sensitivity

(1999)

Multiple Chemical Sensitivity (MCS) is a poorly understood disorder in which a person becomes acutely sensitive to a variety of chemical smells. For some people, the sensitivity began with a toxic exposure, but many patients cannot remember any such exposure. There is now evidence that long-term exposure to *subclinical* levels of toxic substances (e.g., pesticides, exhaust emissions, and air pollutants) can result in sensitivity.

MCS has been studied for over 13 years, and an international consensus process has defined the following symptoms as necessary for diagnosis:

☐ a chronic condition

☐ symptoms recur reproducibly

☐ in response to low levels of exposure

☐ in response to multiple unrelated chemicals

☐ symptoms improve or resolve when incitants are removed

☐ symptoms occur in multiple organ systems

☐ no other single organ disorder can account for the symptoms

Session 1 References

(1999) Multiple Chemical Sensitivity: A Consensus. *Arch.Environ.Health*, 54, 147-149.

Acheson, E.D. (1959). The clinical syndrome variously called benign myalgic encephalomyelitis, Iceland disease and epidemic neurasthaenia. *JAMA*, 26, 569-595.

Bell, D.S. (1995). *The Doctor's Guide to Chronic Fatigue Syndrome,* Boston, MA.

Carruthers, B.M., Jain, A.K., De Meirleir, K., Peterson, D.L., Klimas, N., Lerner, A.M., Bested, A.C., Flor-Henry, P., Joshi, P., Powles, A.C.P., Sherkey, J.A., & van de Sande, M.I. (2003). Myalgic Encephalitis/ Chronic Fatigue Syndrome: Clinical working case definition diagnostic and treatment protocols - A consensus document. Journal of Chronic Fatigue Syndrome 11[1], 7-116.

Carruthers, B.M., van de Sande, M.I., De Meirleir, K.L., Klimas, N.G., Broderick, G., Mitchell, T., Staines, D., Powles, A.P., Speight, N., Vallings, R., Bateman, L., Baumgarten-Austrheim, B., Bell, D.S., Carlo-Stella, N., Chia, J., Darragh, A., Jo, D., Lewis, D., Ligh t, A.R., Marshall-Gradisbik, S., Mena, I., Mikovits, J.A., Miwa, K., Murovska, M., Pall, M.L., & Stevens, S. (2011). Myalgic Encephalomyelitis: International Consensus Criteria. *J Intern.Med.*

Fukuda, K., Straus, S.E., Hickie, I., Sharpe, M.C., Dobbins, J.G., Komaroff, A., & International Chronic Fatigue Syndrome Study Group (1994). The chronic fatigue syndrome: a comprehensive approach to its definition and study. *Annals of Internal Medicine*, 121, 953-959.

Holmes, G.P., Kaplan, J.E., Gantz, N.M., Komaroff, A.L., Schonberger, L.B., Straus, S.E., Jones, J.F., Dubois, R.E., Cunningham-Rundles, C., & Pahwa, S. (1988). Chronic fatigue syndrome: a working case definition. *Annals of Internal Medicine*, 108, 387-389.

Institute of Medicine. (2015). *Beyond Myalgic Encephalomyelitis/Chronic Fatigue Syndrome: Redefining an Illness*. Retrieved from http://www.nap.edu/catalog.php?record_id=19012

Jain, A.K., Carruthers, B.M., van de Sande, M.I., Barron, S.R., Donaldson, C.C., Dunne, J.V., Gingrich, E., Leung, F.I.-K., Malone, D.G., Romano, T.J., Russell, I.J., Saul, D., & Seibel, D.G. (2004). Fibromyalgia Syndrome: Canadian Clinical Working Case Definition, Diagnostic and Treatment Protocols - A Consensus Document. *Journal of Musculoskeletal Pain*, 11, 3- 107.

Jason, L.A., Torres-Harding, S., Jurgens, A., & Helgerson, J. (2004). Comparing the Fukuda et al. Criteria and the Canadian Case Definition for Chronic Fatigue Syndrome. *Journal of Chronic Fatigue Syndrome*, 12, 37-52.

Karnofsky, D.A., Abelmann, W.H., Craver, L.F., & Burchenal, J.H. (1948). The use of the nitrogen mustards in the palliative treatment of carcinoma. *Cancer*, 1, 634-656.

Lorig, K., Halsted, H., Sobel, D., Laurent, D., Gonzalez, V., & Minor, M. (2007). *Living a Healthy Life with Chronic Conditions Canadian Third Edition,* 3rd edn, Bull Publishing, Boulder, Colorado.

Luciano, J.V., Martinez, N., Fernandez-Vergel, R., Garcia-Campayo, J., Verduras, C., Blanco, M.E., Jimenez, M., Ruiz, J.M., Del Hoyo, Y.L., & Serrano-Blanco, A. (2011). Effectiveness of a Psychoeducational Treatment Program Implemented in General Practice for Fibromyalgia Patients: A Randomized Controlled Trial. *Clin J Pain*, 27, 383-391.

Marshall, L., Bested, A., Molot, J., Kerr, K., & Bray, R. (2011). Environmental Sensitivities-Multiple Chemical Sensitivity Status Report. 1-42. Toronto, Canada, Environmental Health Clinic Women's College Hospital, Toronto.

Sears, M.E. (2007). The Medical Perspective on Environmental Sensitivities. 1-79. Ottawa, Canadian Human Rights Commission.

Session 2

Sleep Management

NAVIGATING CHOPPY WATERS

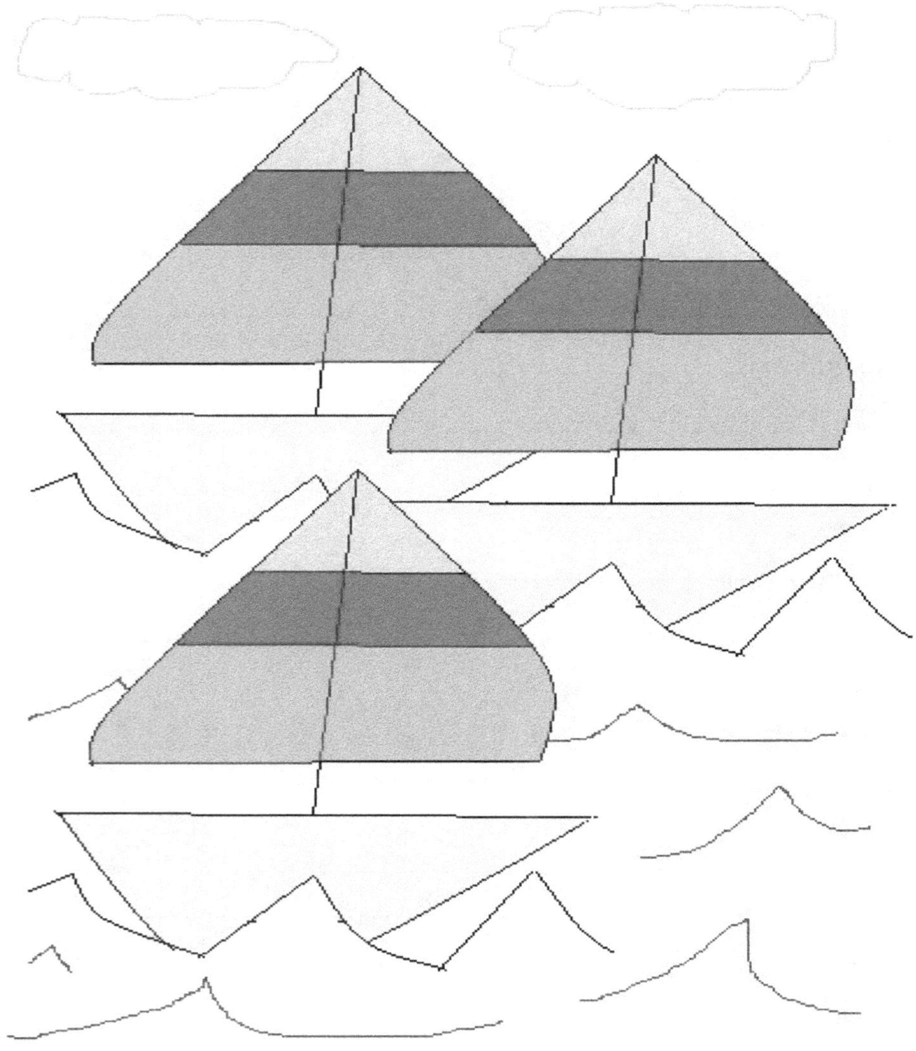

Maureen MacQuarrie, Toronto, ON
(Some thought the waves should be bigger to represent accurately the enormity of the challenges of living with ME/CFS, FM and MCS.)

Session 2

Sleep Management

Objectives

- To increase knowledge about the factors that affect sleep in people with ME/CFS, FM and MCS.
- To improve self-management of sleep.
- To obtain 10 hours of deep, uninterrupted, refreshing sleep per night (or the amount that is right for you).
- To learn to use the *Sleep Chart*.

Before you read on, make sure you have your 2-week baseline Sleep Chart available to refer to.

Sleep Charting

Before reading this section, it is important that you have gathered information about your sleep using the Sleep Chart. Since every day and night is different, charting for at least 2 weeks is necessary to get an accurate idea of typical patterns. You do not have to use the chart recommended in this manual. Any Sleep Chart that includes the following information will be helpful:

- Sleep initiation
- Sleep depth
- Sleep continuation/duration
- Total sleep time
- Total time in bed
- Interferences (e.g., excessive dreaming, restlessness, snoring, external noise, heat, smell, light, etc.)

Normal Sleep

It may be a long time since you slept normally. So, to refresh your memory, the following is what healthy sleep is:

- Healthy people fall asleep in less than 20 minutes without sleep aids, sleep for approximately 7 - 8 hours and wake feeling refreshed.
- Sleep occurs in regular 90-minute cycles of light sleep, then deep sleep, then REM (dreaming sleep). Awakenings occur most often during light and REM sleep or during a change in sleep type (e.g., from REM to light sleep).
- Both sleep duration and sleep depth decrease with age. Infants require several hours per night of deep sleep, whereas healthy elderly individuals may get less than 30 minutes of deep sleep.
- Important hormones such as human growth hormone and melatonin are produced during sleep. Human growth hormone is necessary for tissue repair. And melatonin is necessary for maintaining a stable sleep-wake cycle. Sleep is also critical for the consolidation of memory.

Common Sleep Problems in ME/CFS, FM and MCS

Although many sleep problems are found in ME/CFS and FM (MCS is often associated with severe sleep problems, but has not been formally studied), researchers are still looking for the smoking gun—an objective measure that correlates with morning refreshment and gets better when the patient feels better. The following sleep problems have been measured using sleep EEG in studies of ME/CFS and FM:

- Increased time to fall asleep (sleep latency).
- Increased shifts between sleep stages per hour.
- Decreased deep sleep.
- Decreased sleep time per time spent in bed (sleep efficiency).
- Alpha intrusion into deep sleep (Roizenblatt et al., 2001). This is the intrusion of awake EEG rhythm into deep sleep. Though an objective marker, alpha intrusion is also found in other health conditions associated with disrupted sleep, so cannot be considered diagnostic.
- Increased inspiratory airflow limitations have been reported in the majority of women with FM. This sign is on the spectrum of obstructive sleep apnea, but is not necessarily identifiable by snoring. In one study, a trial of continuous positive airway pressure (CPAP breathing machine) led to decreased daytime symptom scores in over 40% of the subjects (Gold et al., 2004).

A recent area of research that holds promise is in *Cyclic Alternating Pattern* (CAP). Findings have indicated that alpha intrusion is associated with something called Cyclic Alternating Pattern (CAP) on sleep EEG (Rizzi et al., 2004). CAP is, in turn, associated with increased sympathetic drive. Sympathetic drive, also known as *fight or flight*, should be turned down at night so that the body can rest and sleep. This is described in more detail in Session 3 in the section on the *Autonomic Nervous System*. CAP has been found to be elevated in both patients with ME/CFS and FM (Boneva et al., 2007). Furthermore, CAP is associated with poor sleep quality and sleep instability.

A recent but relatively small study by the Toronto sleep physician, Dr. Harvey Moldofsky, has found that in patients whose CAP improved while taking low-dose cyclobenzaprine (a common muscle relaxant which has shown some benefits when used for sleep problems with FM), daytime symptoms such as pain and depression also improved. These findings led Moldofsky and colleagues to wonder if CAP could be a long-sought biological marker for the sleep problems in FM (Moldofsky et al., 2011). The discovery of any reliable biological markers for ME/CFS, FM or MCS will be a big advance, as it will allow physicians to objectively monitor progress and researchers to measure the effectiveness of treatments objectively.

Diagnosing Sleep Problems

Not everyone with ME/CFS, FM and MCS has the same sleep problems. Therefore, the first step in management is to determine what type of sleep problem you have. Use your Sleep Chart to determine if your problems are with falling asleep, staying asleep, oversleeping, and/or unrefreshing sleep. Self-assessment of sleep can be inaccurate. Sometimes people are unaware of falling asleep for short periods, and problems that arise during sleep, such as snoring and sleep apnea, are entirely outside awareness. If you need more accurate information, the following tests can be helpful:

- Home sleep apnea test (level 3 sleep study): This is a test of breathing and blood oxygen saturation (but not including a sleep EEG) that can be done at home. A private company (usually one that sells oxygen and sleep ventilators) will come to your house, teach you how to use the equipment and then return the next day to pick it up. The home test will identify if you snore or stop breathing during sleep and the amount of oxygen in your blood (oxygen saturation) during the night. It does not pick up other types of sleep problems.
- Overnight sleep EEG study (level 1 sleep study): This test, also referred to as polysomnography, is widely available in cities with a medical school or major hospital. The sleep EEG measures a wide range of sleep-related disorders, including limb movements, narcolepsy, sleep apneas, and whether you have alpha intrusion (found in ME/CFS and FM).

Many American physicians are on record as recommending a sleep study for all patients with ME/CFS or FM, as the rate of picking up some treatable problem (e.g., sleep apnea) is over 20%. If the alpha intrusion and CAP are measured, which they often are not, the rate of abnormal studies is likely much higher.

If your sleep is unrefreshing and your physician recommends a sleep study, it is worth your time to find out which sleep clinic near you has the most interest or expertise in the sleep problems found in ME/CFS or FM. In clinics run by respiratory physicians (those interested in breathing), many of the interesting findings in patients with ME/CFS and FM may be overlooked. As mentioned earlier, these include, but are not limited to, alpha intrusion, decreased sleep efficiency, and increased inspiratory pressures.

I have been repeatedly surprised by sleep study findings. It's very hard to assess during an office visit whether a sleep problem that may be diagnosed by a sleep study exists. If in doubt, check it out (i.e., go for the study). It would be very disconcerting if, after months or years of self-management, you found out that you had sleep apnea, instead of ME/CFS and that it was treatable with a ventilator. There are a number of people who have ME/CFS, FM and/or MCS in addition to sleep apnea. Treating the sleep apnea may help, but will not cure the other conditions.

Joan's Sleep Chart

While reading this section, have Joan's Sleep Chart and your own in front of you to refer to. Do you notice any similarities or differences between your Sleep Chart and Joan's? If so, some of the suggestions below may be of help to you.

Joan often has problems falling asleep, some days worse than others. She almost always wakes unrefreshed. As noted earlier, use your Sleep Chart to determine if your problems are with falling asleep, staying asleep, oversleeping, or unrefreshing sleep.

From Joan's Sleep Chart, we can see that Joan's energy and pain vary day-to-day. In terms of prognosis, this is a good sign. It means that if she can figure out what causes her symptoms to fluctuate, she may be able to improve her sleep and, as a result, have better and more consistent health.

Joan's energy remains fairly stable on the days after she works. This suggests that she is able to work sustainably at the level of 2 X 4-hour shifts per week. Eating out may be a problem. It took Joan a particularly long time to fall asleep the night after she went out to dinner with friends. This will be something Joan will have to observe further. Is this typical for her after a meal out? If so, is it due to the change in her routine, or could it be related to what she ate? Then again, the insomnia could have been caused by exposure to personal fragrances or other chemicals in the restaurant.

To determine which of these possibilities is the most likely, Joan will need to go out for dinner a few more times. She will need to keep track of the possible variables and see if a pattern emerges. For example, if she has insomnia only sometimes when she goes out, then it isn't likely that the disruption to her schedule is the cause. It must be something specific about an individual outing.

Walking increases Joan's pain the following day, but doesn't decrease her energy. Keep this in mind when we get to Session 3 on Activity and Exercise. Since exercise doesn't reliably cause Joan to feel worse with respect to energy, she fits better into the diagnostic category of FM than ME/CFS. Post-exertional malaise is a mandatory criterion of ME/CFS. It's tricky, though, since the reaction can be delayed.

Since Joan is able to tolerate exercise from an energy perspective (i.e., her energy doesn't decline when she exercises), she may be able to find an activity that will allow her to increase her stamina and fitness. Joan might benefit from a gym or water-based program that doesn't stress the injured ankle. On the other hand, more regular exercise may result in increased pain and decreased energy. She will only find this out by trying different exercise routines.

For each rating of energy and pain, Joan then plotted her scores on the graph at the bottom of the Sleep Chart. She used different colours so that patterns would become apparent. You can see that there are some mirror images apparent between energy and pain; when energy is higher, pain is lower and vice versa. This suggests that in Joan's case, the two symptoms are related. As mentioned in the Introduction, this means that if Joan can figure out a way to improve one of these symptoms, the other may also improve.

The Sleep Chart is showing Joan more than simply her sleep patterns. By studying it, Joan can start to see some useful interconnections between sleep, energy, and pain. In the remainder of this session, we will be looking more closely at sleep and some steps that can be taken to improve it. Joan already understands that it is only one part of the whole picture. She is also beginning to understand that what she does during the day has an impact on her sleep.

Remember that it is useful to establish your baseline (a good idea of your personal symptom patterns) BEFORE you make any changes. To determine her baseline, Joan kept her bedtime medications the same every day and didn't make any changes to her nutritional supplements during this first two weeks. There is no magic time required to find your baseline; two weeks may be sufficient, or you may need to chart for a month or longer to be satisfied you have a sense of how your sleep, pain, and energy are interrelated.

Once you are satisfied that you have established a baseline, you are ready to start thinking about behavioral changes to improve your sleep. To assist you in analyzing your baseline information, I strongly recommend plotting the values from the top of your Sleep Chart onto the graph at the bottom as Joan did. Also, using a different color for each symptom is invaluable. Even while making the charts for this manual, I became confused with the charts and added texture so that the black and white printed lines could be distinguished from each other.

Joan plotted both energy and pain and was able to notice a relationship between the two symptoms. See if you can identify any patterns, such as Joan has found. Are there things you are doing that might be triggering sleep issues?

Improving Sleep: Behavioral Change

The most successful remedy for sleep problems in general is to change behavior. Our bodies rely on signals from the environment, such as sunlight, and our habitual behaviors to tell them when it's time to sleep and when it's time to wake up. If we keep unpredictable hours and activity patterns, our bodies will be confused. If we keep a routine, our bodies will form "good" habits.

The behaviors that help us form these good habits are called *sleep hygiene*. There are several excellent books outlining the basics of sleep hygiene. *No More Sleepless Nights* by Peter Hauri and *Say Goodnight to Insomnia* by Gregg Jacobs are two good ones. In my opinion, for patients with severe sleep problems, these sleep hygiene strategies are necessary (and without them, other interventions such as medication will not work well), but they are often not sufficient. In other words, the other interventions are also needed.

The five categories below all form part of good sleep hygiene:

1. Setting the Stage

- Identify your natural sleep window (i.e., when do you usually go to sleep, and when do you usually wake up?)
- Keep a regular routine, especially your wake-up time, so that your body gets in the habit of sleeping and waking at consistent times.
- Start your sleep time routine (e.g., meditation, hot bath, snack) about one hour before your ideal sleep time.

2. Identify and Eliminate Factors That Interfere With Sleep

- In patients with ME/CFS especially, activity in excess of energy levels results in increased adrenaline. This is identifiable by an increased heart rate and the feeling of being "tired but wired." Pacing, which we investigate in Session 3, will decrease this problem.

- Avoid the use of stimulants (e.g., coffee, chocolate).
- Some over-the-counter cold remedies contain stimulant decongestants such as phenylephrine. These should be avoided.
- Exposure to food or chemicals to which a person is sensitive can result in disrupted sleep. This can only be identified by careful observation since the triggers are different for each person. More about this in Session 6.
- Stress and anxiety are common causes of sleep problems. Encourage yourself to set a time in the day to problem-solve and then let the problems go until the next day. Staying up worrying is counterproductive since if you don't sleep well, you will be less able to problem-solve the next day.
- Daytime naps (i.e., actually sleeping) are generally problematic for nighttime sleep. Resting (without sleeping) is recommended for those patients who find it helpful. However, some severely ill individuals require a sleeping nap to prevent extreme exhaustion. Extreme exhaustion can be accompanied by an increase in adrenaline levels. This increase makes nighttime sleeping more difficult and should be avoided. You will have to experiment with both resting and napping to see the effects of each. Don't underestimate the value of a horizontal rest in the day.
- Exposure to bright light before bed from watching TV, using the computer, or reading blocks the production of melatonin and should be avoided.

3. Practice Good Sleep Hygiene

- Use the bedroom only for sleep and sex.
- If you don't sleep after 15 – 20 minutes, get out of bed. This is a tricky recommendation for people who are too exhausted to get out of bed. Use your judgment.
- Don't go to bed until you are tired.
- Sleep restriction is a common behavioral strategy for insomnia and disrupted sleep. At first glance, it sounds like torture...to purposely stay up late even when one is exhausted. The rationale for sleep restriction is to train the body to fall asleep when it is really tired (ideally without medication) and sleep soundly for a shorter time rather than lying in bed tossing and turning for a longer period of time.

  The boxes below and on the next page contain a summary of the instructions for sleep restriction used by the Calgary Chronic Pain Centre. These instructions are provided with permission from the author.

The following four steps for Sleep Restriction are recommended by the Calgary Chronic Pain Centre and are summarized here with permission from the author (Currie & Wilson, 2002; Currie et al., 2000):

Step 1. Look at your Sleep Chart and calculate your average **Sleep Efficiency** for the previous week. Sleep Efficiency = hours asleep divided by hours in bed X 100%. For example, if you were in bed 8 hours but asleep only 4 hours, your efficiency would be 50% (4 ÷ 8 x 100). The goal of sleep restriction is to increase sleep efficiency to above 85%. If your sleep efficiency is already above 85%, STOP now; you don't have to continue with the rest of the steps. Some people with ME/CFS and FM (rarer with MCS) are hypersomniac, meaning they sleep more than the normal 7-8 hours/night. These people shouldn't engage in sleep restriction unless they also spend a lot of time in bed not sleeping.

Step 2. Calculate your average **Total Sleep Time** per night for the past week and determine when you get your best sleep. Use this information to set your sleep window (which will be explained in Step 3) for the coming week.

Step 3. Starting with tonight, **restrict the amount of time you spend in bed to the value of your average total sleep time.** It is best to do this by going to bed later at night rather than getting up earlier in the morning. For example, if your average total sleep time was 4½ hours and you normally get up at 7 am, you will need to adjust your bedtime to 2:30 am. When you are trying to improve your sleep efficiency and quality, you should get up at the same time each morning. This may involve several alarm clocks since you might just be getting too deep into sleep when your sleep window ends. Therefore, your sleep window is the 4½ hours between 2:30 am and 7 am. Maintain this sleep window until your sleep efficiency reaches the target of 85%.

NOTE: **Never go below 4 hours for your sleep window.** If your average nightly total sleep time is less than this amount, then use 4 hours as your starting sleep window.

Step 4. Gradually (weekly or every two weeks) add 15 minutes to your sleep window (usually by an earlier bedtime) until your average sleep efficiency is 85% or greater (target level) **and** you have reached a total sleep time that allows you to wake refreshed.

Don't add 15 minutes until you have followed the sleep restriction guidelines for 1 - 2 weeks and have begun to notice some improvement (e.g., fewer awakenings or falling asleep faster).

Instructions continued on the next page.

Sleep Restriction instructions (continued).

Follow a schedule of gradual increases to the sleep window. For example, if a 1-week increase of 15 minutes leads to maintenance or continued improvements from the previous week, add another 15 minutes the following week. However, if an increase leads to a decrease in sleep efficiency (i.e., you spend the extra time tossing and turning instead of sleeping), go back to the previous sleep times until you see improvements again.

Continue to use the Sleep Chart to note your progress. As long as your sleep efficiency is at your target level, continue to gradually increase your sleep window until you have reached a total sleep time that you are comfortable with. Keep up this final night's pattern.

4. Improve the Sleep Environment

- Eyeshades (available at local pharmacies) and blackout blinds are essential so that your body realizes it is night and gets ready to sleep by producing melatonin. Even a small amount of light will stop the production of melatonin. Melatonin is a critical hormone for sleep. Please note that melatonin production is also thought to be impaired by exposure to electrical current during the night (e.g., from a clock radio, bedside light, or alarm clock).
- A comfortable bed is important, especially if pain is an issue. Usually, a firm mattress, to allow movement and change of position, with a pillow top, to decrease pressure points, works best. "Egg carton" foam or a padded cover can be purchased and is cheaper than buying a new mattress. People with MCS are unlikely to tolerate the off-gassing from new foam and may have to manage with an older mattress or purchase one with natural fibres at greater cost.
- The most effective earplugs are the beeswax or silicone types sold at many pharmacies and online. Foam and plastic are much less comfortable and are ineffective.
- Custom earplugs (much more expensive) cut out over 80% of all noise and don't fall out during the night. They are typically available through audiologists. Please be aware that if you are a side sleeper, the harder custom earplugs may cause pressure and pain on the ear cartilage.
- If you have a sleeping partner who is very restless or snores loudly, a trial of sleeping apart may be helpful to determine if your partner is adding to your sleep problems. Maybe your partner could benefit from a sleep assessment. This is a frequent prescription in my office.

5. Diet Considerations

- Sleep can be significantly affected by the food you eat. How to determine the effects of individual foods will be discussed in the session on diet (Session 5).
- Some people with ME/CFS, FM and MCS have symptoms that may be related to blood sugar fluctuations (this has never been proven). Some people sleep better on an empty stomach, while others sleep better after eating a carbohydrate or protein snack. You will have to experiment to see what works best for you. Be wary of having the same snack every night. Foods you especially crave are likely to be those that are causing symptoms.

As I already mentioned, for most patients with ME/CFS, FM and MCS, these changes alone are necessary but insufficient to restore healthy sleep and medications must also be used.

Natural Sleep Remedies

Please note this is not an exhaustive list of sleep remedies or their benefits and side effects. Please collaborate with a licensed health care professional when trying these products. Even though they can be purchased over the counter, natural health products can interact with other drugs and supplements and can cause harm.

Melatonin

- Melatonin is a naturally produced hormone, a byproduct of tryptophan. It is produced by the pineal gland during deep sleep and in the skin with exposure to infrared light from the sun. It is possible to test saliva melatonin levels to see whether you are producing enough.
- Melatonin is critical in maintaining circadian rhythm, when you wake and fall asleep.
- Oral melatonin (1 - 3 mg) helps restore your normal sleep schedule after disruption from jet lag or shift work.
- Melatonin should be taken 2 - 3 hours prior to the hoped-for sleep time (i.e., NOT at bedtime) to be effective.
- Melatonin is effective in changing and stabilizing the sleep/wake cycle. In ME/CFS, FM and MCS and in shift workers and travellers, melatonin helps stabilize the sleep-wake cycle. This is helpful for people with irregular sleep times or whose sleep window creeps later and later (i.e., preventing creep). The benefits of melatonin are augmented by adding bright light therapy in the morning.
- Subsequent to the first edition of this manual, research has been published suggesting that melatonin is also useful for insomnia, especially in the elderly (Auld, Maschauer, Morrison, Skene, & Riha, 2017). It decreases the amount of time it takes to get to sleep.

Magnesium

- Taken approx. one hour before bedtime, magnesium (Mg) acts as a mild nerve and muscle relaxant.
- The recommended dose ranges from 250 mg to 1.5 g, depending on bowel tolerance. Too much Mg will cause diarrhea. In this case, just cut back the dose slightly until you get the desired effect without the side effects.

L-Theanine

- L-Theanine before bed is reported to increase alpha EEG rhythm (relaxed awake state). It may help reduce stress-induced "excitation" and help people become ready for sleep. It does not appear to actually put people to sleep.
- The recommended dose is 200 mg, up to three times daily. When taken during the day, L-theanine can ease feelings of anxiety. (I also suggest it for this purpose). Theanine can be measured as part of a urine amino acid panel (See Session 9 for more on this test).

5-HTP

- 5-HTP is the immediate precursor of serotonin. Serotonin is necessary for deep sleep and many other homeostatic functions, such as eating and temperature. Many sleep protocols recommend 5-HTP, though the research supporting its use is sparse. There are widely varying recommended doses. When used to help with depression, 5-HTP should be used three times daily. For sleep, use approximately 50 - 100 mg before bed.
- 5-HTP may help improve parasympathetic tone. The parasympathetic branch of the autonomic nervous system is responsible for calming after a fight or flight response. Parasympathetic tone is decreased in most people with ME/CFS and FM as tested by heart rate variability analysis. See Session 3 for more on the autonomic nervous system.
- **CAUTION:** 5-HTP should **NOT** be used, or used with extreme caution, in people on antidepressants that increase serotonin levels. Such drugs include amitriptyline (Elavil®), fluoxetine (Prozac®) and all other Selective Serotonin Reuptake Inhibitors (SSRIs), mirtazapine (Remeron®), and selegiline. Using 5-HTP with one of these drugs can cause the dangerous serotonin syndrome (symptoms include: agitation, increased muscle tone, increased temperature). Use this supplement only under supervision from your physician. This is a reminder that natural is not synonymous with safe.

Fatigued to Fantastic® Sleep Formula

This sleep formula is part of Dr. Jacob Teitelbaum's Fatigued to Fantastic program.The supplement contains

- Valerian (Valeriana officinalis) 200 mg

- Passionflower (Passiflora incarnata) 90 mg
- L-Theanine (Suntheanine® brand) 50 mg
- Hops (Humulus lupulus) Flower Extract 30 mg
- Wild Lettuce (Lactuca virosa) Leaf Extract 18 mg
- Jamaica Dogwood (Piscidia piscipula) 12 mg
- Wild Lettuce (Lactuca virosa) Leaf 10 mg

Note: Many sensitive individuals are unable to tolerate mixtures of several compounds. The risk of being intolerant to a product varies with the number of ingredients.

Hypnotic (Sleep-Inducing) Medications

Despite disciplined sleep hygiene and use of natural products, many, if not most, patients with ME/CFS, FM and MCS require sleep medication to get the sleep required to function. Some people's ability to sleep is so disrupted that they cannot sleep at all without medication.

Many patients and physicians are opposed, in principle, to the use of sleep medications for longer than a couple of weeks. This principle is based on the serious side effects that accompanied the use of older sleep remedies. Newer medications have fewer risks; however, any medication that promotes sleep may overshoot and cause a "hangover" in the morning by lasting longer than anticipated.

Whenever trying a new medication, try it first on a weekend day and notice when the effects wear off for you. Then try taking it that many hours before you need to be awake and see if you can find a window in which the benefits outweigh the risks. When doing this assessment, remember to compare the risk of chronic under-sleep to the risk involved in taking the medication. Chronic under-sleep is associated with increased incidence of traffic accidents, decreased memory and cognitive function, and increased risk of overweight and heart disease. Many sleep medications have similar side effects. Of course, you will have to weigh the risks and benefits with your physician since any of these next suggestions require a prescription.

Keep in mind the following:

- Start LOW and go SLOW with all medication trials.
- No one drug will improve all sleep parameters. Most patients have to take a combination of medications (e.g., one to fall asleep and one to stay asleep).

- Be aware that although the medications mentioned below are generally safe and well-tolerated, any medication can have serious adverse effects in sensitive patients.
- Be cautious with any medication trial and always consult with your family doctor to ensure a medication will not have a unique adverse effect because of your unique health history or other medications you are taking.
- Some patients develop tolerance to sleep medications and have to rotate/switch medications every few months to maintain the desired effect. Physicians are generally unfamiliar with the strategy of rotating sleep medications, but they may have heard of rotating pain medications to diminish tolerance. This is the same principle; rotation generally results in patients using less medication since the rotation decreases tolerance and thus lower doses will be effective. It may not work for everyone. Be prepared that some trials will be unsuccessful.
- What follows is not an exhaustive list of all the sleep medications and their potential side effects. Obtain more information from your physician and pharmacist to ensure you are fully informed.

Zopiclone (Imovane®)

- Decreases sleep initiation.
- The average required dose is higher in patients with more severe sleep disruption and more severe illness.
- Many physicians hold the false belief that zopiclone is addictive or that tolerance will develop. However, the authoritative textbook on pharmacology, Goodman and Gilman's *The Pharmacological Basis of Therapeutics,* states that this fear has no basis in reality and that the Z drug family (of which zopiclone is a member) can be used for long-term sleep problems (2001).
- Some patients with MCS may require very low doses (i.e., less than one tablet), but most patients will require 5 - 15 mg at bedtime. Always take zopiclone as you turn out the light. It works quickly, and if you are not ready to sleep, you may miss the height of the effect.
- Zopiclone only lasts 3 - 4 hours. Therefore, many patients who require the drug to sleep will wake up after this period of time and require a "split dose." A split dose is an additional dose typically equal to 1/2 of the dose initially required to get to sleep.
- Zopiclone can leave an unpleasant taste in the mouth. It can also cause nausea, agitation, or hangover symptoms in sensitive individuals. There are reports of abnormal behaviors such as overeating in people taking zopiclone. Be on the lookout for signs of this.

L-Tryptophan (Tryptan®)

- Is a naturally occurring substance—an amino acid found in most complete proteins, such as meat.

- Research using sleep study data is mixed in terms of the effectiveness of L-tryptophan for improving sleep.
- Due to side effects caused by processing impurities several years ago, tryptophan fell into disfavor. However, the problems in the manufacturing of tryptophan have been corrected, and there have been no reports of serious side effects for many years. As a result of this history, in Canada, L-Tryptophan was temporarily available only by prescription.
- The effective dose for sleep initiation varies from 500 mg to 5000 mg. Higher doses are also used as an adjunct for depression.
- Tryptophan has a short duration of action (2 - 4 hours), and a split dose upon awaking in the middle of the night may be necessary.
- Approximately 10% of patients have a "paradoxical" reaction to tryptophan. In these individuals, tryptophan causes alertness instead of sedation. This may be due to a pathway that converts tryptophan into quinolinic acid, a substance that is toxic to the brain. People with this paradoxical effect should avoid using L-tryptophan and try 5-HTP instead. 5-HTP, like tryptophan, is a precursor to serotonin. Unlike L-tryptophan, 5-HTP does not get metabolized to quinolinic acid.

Test: Quinolinic acid can be measured as part of a urine organic acid panel (OAT panel)
Available: Mosaic Diagnostics (https://mosaicdx.com/)

- **CAUTION:** Like 5-HTP, tryptophan can lead to serotonin syndrome if used in conjunction with a serotonin antidepressant such as amitriptyline (Elavil®), fluoxetine (Prozac®) and all other selective serotonin reuptake inhibitors (SSRIs), mirtazapine (Remeron®), and selegiline.

Amitriptyline (Elavil®)

- Helps increase the duration of sleep and decreases awakenings. May help with sleep initiation.
- Amitriptyline is a tricyclic antidepressant (TCA). In low doses, TCAs have been an effective treatment for sleep and pain in people with fibromyalgia and other chronic pain conditions. More research has been done on the tricyclics for this use than on any other drug class.
- The effective antidepressant dose of TCAs ranges from 75 - 250 mg/day. In patients with ME/CFS, FM and MCS, the effective dose for sleep improvement ranges from 10 - 50 mg before bed. Even at this dose, some sensitive patients will experience too many side effects to continue use. Some professionals in the field recommend starting with a 2 mg dose. This requires a compounding pharmacy to make up capsules since the smallest commercially available dose is 10 mg.

- The onset of TCAs can be slow, especially in people with poor digestive function. Therefore, take this drug 1 - 2 hours before the intended sleep time and notice for yourself the time between taking the drug and the onset of action so that you can time it to your best advantage.
- Amitriptyline shares side effects with all drugs in its class. These include dry mouth, increased heart rate, dizziness when standing, constipation, weight gain, morning hangover, and difficulty focusing the eyes on close objects.

Trazodone (Desyrel®)

- Trazodone is an antidepressant that improves sleep initiation and duration.
- 25 - 100 mg is taken 1/2 hour or more before bedtime.
- Trazodone has fewer side effects than amitriptyline; it does not cause dry mouth or increased heart rate.
- Trazodone does not have a beneficial effect on pain.

Clonazepam (Rivotril®)

- Benzodiazepines are NOT recommended as a long-term sleep aid. This is because of the development of tolerance (decreased benefit over time) and withdrawal (difficulty discontinuing the drug after prolonged use).
- However, in selected patients with physical restlessness and pain caused by painful muscle spasms, clonazepam can help in a way that no other drug can.
- Clonazepam is also helpful for some patients whose anxiety symptoms prevent them from sleeping.
- Clonazepam has a preferable side effect profile in terms of tolerance and tendency to be overused compared to other benzodiazepines such as lorazepam and alprazolam.

Quetiapine (Seroquel®)

- This drug is a newer antipsychotic drug (called an atypical antipsychotic) and is often used for severe anxiety.
- Patients with ME/CFS, FM and MCS with significant anxiety, which has not responded to other treatments, and which is interfering with sleep, may benefit from this drug at small doses.
- Weight gain and daytime sedation are the primary side effects, and they can be severe.
- A few of my patients have had severe cognitive side effects from this drug. Therefore, I always start with very cautious doses of 12.5 - 25 mg and work up. The antipsychotic dose for this drug is up to 800 mg/day. However, few ME/CFS, FM or MCS patients would tolerate that dose.

Pregabalin (Lyrica®)

- This is a drug used primarily for chronic neuropathic pain. It has also been approved for use in fibromyalgia.
- In my experience, pregabalin is the most effective drug for other neuropathic pain syndromes, but its effect in FM is variable.
- There is some preliminary evidence that pregabalin increases deep sleep. If this is true, this would be one of the very few drugs that does this. Some of my patients with severe sleep problems have used pregabalin with good effect for this off-label use. Others have felt too dopey on it even at the lowest dose.
- Side effects include cognitive blunting, daytime fatigue, swelling, and weight gain, which can be limiting in some patients.
- Gabapentin (Neurontin®), another drug used in neuropathic pain, also has sedating side effects that are helpful for some patients.

Mirtazapine (Remeron®)

- This is a newer antidepressant that works on serotonin but uses a different mechanism than other SSRIs such as fluoxetine (Prozac®).
- I have found it very useful for both depression and severe anxiety. Sedation is a side effect of this drug and can be profound. For some, this can be helpful in terms of falling asleep and sleeping longer. For others, mirtazapine causes too much daytime sedation to be useful.
- The sleep effect with mirtazapine is better at lower doses (15 – 30 mg) as opposed to the higher doses that are often used for depression and anxiety (40 – 60 mg). More is not always better.
- Tolerance to the hypnotic (sleep) effect of mirtazapine develops quickly. It works best if not used every night.

Lemborexant (Dayvigo®) and Daridorexant (Quviviq®)

- Dual orexin receptor antagonist (DORA) drugs were introduced in 2014. They block orexin, a brain chemical responsible for wakefulness. Orexin neurons occur only in the brain, so there may be fewer side effects than when using medications with receptors throughout the body (Kishi et al., 2021).
- A review of studies of lemborexant suggests it improves total sleep time, waking after sleep onset and sleep efficiency (Waters, 2021). The amount of the drug in the body decreases to about ¼ the effective dose by morning, and in the nine studies to date, there is no evidence of impaired cognitive function or increased risk of falls.

- People report better morning alertness with lemborexant than with a placebo—possibly because the drug improved sleep quality.
- DORA drugs don't act on the GABA or histamine and so may not carry the feared increased risk of dementia that accompanies most other sleeping medications.

Tetrahydrocannabinol (THC) and Cannabidiol (CBD)

Now that naturally occurring cannabinoids are legally accessible in most countries, sales of synthetic products have plummeted. People clearly prefer natural cannabis products.

- An extensive review of the health effects of cannabis and cannabinoids by the National Academy of Medicine in the U.S. concludes that there is moderate evidence that cannabinoids improve sleep quality and daytime refreshment in people with fibromyalgia and chronic pain (National Academies of Sciences & Medicine, 2017). However, the research is hampered by the lack of comparison of different strains and cannabis molecules and mode of delivery (e.g., oral, inhalation or vaping).
- It is important to be aware that, although naturally occurring, cannabis has side effects. Some side effects, like getting high or getting the munchies, are not too serious. Some are more problematic, such as an increased risk of psychosis in younger and heavy users. Cannabis is not recommended at all for people under the age of 25.
- Some studies show that cannabis worsens sleep quality (Choi, Huang, & Gamaldo, 2020).
- Tolerance develops to the sleep effects of cannabis. This means that over time, people may need to increase the dose to get the same effect, and when people discontinue cannabis, they often experience insomnia for a period. This can make it hard for people to discontinue use when they wish.
- Given the number of cannabis products available and significant individual variation in response, I recommend consulting a knowledgeable professional to help you make an informed decision.

Do Sleep Medications Increase the Risk of Dementia?

There is a concern that sleep medications, especially the benzodiazepines (like Xanax®, Ativan® and others) and possibly the Z-drugs like zopiclone (Imovane® & Zimovane®) and zolpidem (Sublinox® & Ambien®), increase the risk of dementia when used over time. This concern is based on a flurry of population-based studies in the mid-2010s. A review of 11 of these studies concluded that regular benzodiazepine use increases risk of dementia, perhaps by as much as 50% (Pariente, de Gage, Moore, & Bégaud, 2016). Since dementia is a common condition, a 50% increase is alarming.

Research on dementia risk is difficult to conduct. For ethical reasons, one can't purposely give a drug to participants that may have adverse effects to study what happens. Therefore, the studies connecting sleep medication and dementia are observational—seeing whether people who are using the sleep drugs are more likely to develop dementia than those who are not. However compelling, it is an error to assume there is a causal connection, i.e., that the drugs cause dementia.

More recent research refutes the earlier findings, concluding that there is "no causal effect of benzodiazepines or Z-drugs on dementia incidence." (Richardson et al., 2019). In a 2024 study that included brain imaging, there was a small association between benzodiazepine use and smaller hippocampal volume. The hippocampus is critical to memory. However, the association was not dose-dependent (people taking more medication did not have a bigger decrease in hippocampal size), and there was no correlation between drug use and dementia (Hofe et al., 2024).

The more recent research suggests that the fears arising from earlier research may be unfounded. Nevertheless, it is always better to use natural means to achieve sleep if possible. Medications can make people unconscious and unaware, but this state does not mimic natural sleep.

Preparing for Session 3

Before reading this session, it is strongly recommended that you spend 2 weeks getting to know and recording your activity level. You may, if you choose, continue to use the Sleep Chart daily during this time. But if you find this too draining on your energy, only do the charting recommended in each session. Find the balance that is right for you.

If you are working through this program on your own, you can do so at the pace that works for your particular concerns. Perhaps you'd like to concentrate on sleep for a while. If so, continue charting using the Sleep Chart so that you can measure if the changes you make have any effect. Once you are ready, and before you move on to Session 3, spend 2 weeks charting your activity levels.

To do the charting in the same way that Joan did, you will need the following:

- Activity Log
- Adapted Karnofsky Energy Rating Scale
- Sleep Chart (which Joan uses only to plot her Energy/Functional Capacity levels)

Joan's Activity Log

The Activity Log is a way to visualize the pattern of your daily activities. Joan divided her activities into four categories and coloured each one a different colour so that she could easily see her daily activity patterns. For this chart, sleeping is not considered "an activity," and Joan's sleep times are left blank (white). Joan chose the following categories:

- Rest/Crash includes intentional rest time and the time during which Joan is too tired to accomplish anything but is not asleep (orange). This includes couch and TV time, but not reading or using the computer.
- Low Activity/Puttering includes moving around, doing necessary habitual activities that don't require much thought or energy (purple).
- Physical Activity, for Joan, includes walking the dog, showering and heavier housework (green); for you, this may be a bit different.
- Focused Activity refers to tasks that require mental concentration, such as talking to others, driving, doing errands, emailing, and reading (pink).

You may choose different activity categories. The objective here is to identify how you spend your day and how you split up activities of a similar nature. Take a day or two to decide what activity categories make sense for you.

- Using the Adapted Karnofsky Energy Rating Scale, Joan rated her energy when she got up each morning and again before bed.
- She also recorded the number of hours of sleep each night. The number of sleep hours is less than the number of hours she was in bed, as she usually wakes up one or more times over the course of the night.
- Joan recorded the number of "usable hours/day." She did this by adding the time spent in *activities/ exercise* (coloured green on the graph) and *focused activities* (coloured pink on the graph).
- She did not include the time spent resting, crashed or the time spent doing activities that didn't require physical or mental concentration.
- Usable hours/day is a way of estimating how many hours you would be able to work inside or outside the home and accomplish useful or remunerative tasks.
- Therefore, puttering and couch time are not included in the calculation of usable hours per day. Joan only did one week of the Activity Log. I am asking that you do two.

physical activity — low activity — crashed but awake — focussed activity

Activity Log

Name: Joan Smith Date: Dec 26/11

Day	Monday	Tuesday	Wednesday	Thursday	Friday	Saturday	Sunday
No. of Hrs. Sleep ~~1:00am–8:00am~~	7.5	7.0	8.0	6.5	8.0	7.5	9.0
Sleep Quality		1 = very poor	2 = poor	3 = fair	4 = good	5 = very good	
Functional Capacity Scale at beginning of day 0 – 10 (see reverse)	6	5	5	5.5	6	6.5	4
Activities (please specify)							
8:00 am				wake up get ready			
9:00 am	wake up	wake up	wake up	eat	wake up get ready	wake up eat	
10:00 am	eat get ready	get up	eat	work		dog walk	
11:00 am	dog walk shower		dog walk		dog walk shower	shopping + coffee	wake up
12:00 pm	pick up parents	dog walk	errands with parents		lunch with friend		uggh
1:00 pm		groceries	doctor			cook + organize	eat
2:00 pm	boxing day with family	clean kitchen	bank			lunch	walk + bathe dog
3:00 pm				rest	doctor's appt.		
4:00 pm	big dinner	rest	eat	walk dog	paper work	rest	laundry
5:00 pm		talk phone	phone / email	clean cook	dinner	dinner with friend	phone
6:00 pm		dinner	computer	dinner, phone / emails	cleaning		dinner
7:00 pm	home		couch with dog				shower
8:00 pm		couch			couch		
9:00 pm	couch		snack	couch		NYE	couch
10:00 pm	bed	bed	bed		bed		
11:00 pm				bed		home	bed
12:00 am							
1:00 am						bed	
No. of Mins. Walked / Day	15	10	20	20	15	15	15
No. of Usable Hours / Day	9.5	6	8	9.5	9	12	5.5
Functional Capacity Scale at end of day 0 – 10 (see reverse)	4	3	3.5	3	4	4	3

Joan's Sleep Chart (for activity)

- To determine whether her daily energy was stable, Joan also charted her morning and afternoon energy levels using the graph on the Sleep Chart.
- These are the same values noted in the two Functional Capacity rows of the Activity Log, but as you will see, charting them on the Sleep Chart allows one to easily note the changes in energy from the beginning to the end of the day.
- Joan connected the morning and evening energy ratings with a line to see whether she was maintaining or losing energy each day. She noticed that she had a consistent pattern of downward arrows.

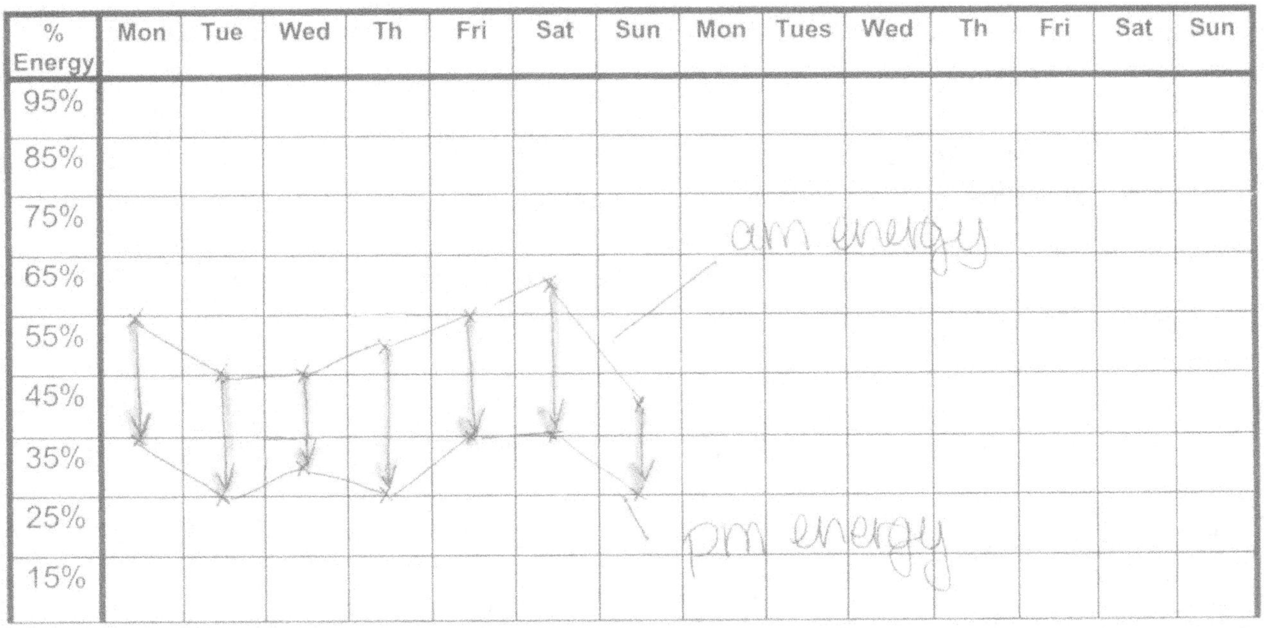

Adapted from the "sleep sheet" of Dr. Beverley Tompkins, Burke Institute, Calgary

Session 2 References

(2001) *Goodman & Gillman's The pharmacological basis of therapeutics,* Tenth Edition, McGraw-Hill.

Auld, F., Maschauer, E. L., Morrison, I., Skene, D. J., & Riha, R. L. (2017). Evidence for the efficacy of melatonin in the treatment of primary adult sleep disorders. *Sleep Medicine Reviews, 34*, 10–22. doi:https://doi.org/10.1016/j.smrv.2016.06.005

Boneva, R.S., Decker, M.J., Maloney, E.M., Lin, J.M., Jones, J.F., Helgason, H.G., Heim, C.M., Rye, D.B., & Reeves, W.C. (2007). Higher heart rate and reduced heart rate variability persist during sleep in chronic fatigue syndrome: A population-based study 1. *Auton.Neurosci.*, 137, 94-101.

Choi, S., Huang, B. C., & Gamaldo, C. E. (2020). Therapeutic Uses of Cannabis on Sleep Disorders and Related Conditions. *Journal of Clinical Neurophysiology, 37*(1), 39–49. doi:https://dx.doi.org/10.1097/WNP.0000000000000617

Currie, S.R. & Wilson, K.G. (2002). *60 Second Sleep Ease: Quick Tips to Get a Good Night's Rest,* New Horizon Press, New Jersey.

Currie, S.R., Wilson, K.G., Pontefract, A.J., & deLaplante, L. (2000). Cognitive and Behavioral Treatment of Insomnia Secondary to Chronic Pain. *Journal of Consulting and Clinical Psychology*, 68, 407-416.

Gold, A.R., Dipalo, F., Gold, M.S., & Broderick, J. (2004). Inspiratory airflow dynamics during sleep in women with fibromyalgia. *Sleep*, 27, 459-466.

Hofe, I.V., Stricker, B.H., Vernooij, M.W., Ikram, M.K., Ikram, M.A., & Wolters, F.J. (2024). Benzodiazepine use in relation to long-term dementia risk and imaging markers of neurodegeneration: a population-based study. *BMC medicine, 22*(1), 266. doi:https://pubmed.ncbi.nlm.nih.gov/38951846/

Kishi, T., Nishida, M., Koebis, M., Taninaga, T., Muramoto, K., Kubota, N., . . . Iwata, N. (2021). Evidence-based insomnia treatment strategy using novel orexin antagonists: A review. *Neuropsychopharmacology Reports, 23*, 23. doi:https://dx.doi.org/10.1002/npr2.12205

Moldofsky, H., Harris, H.W., Archambault, W.T., Kwong, T., & Lederman, S. (2011). Effects of bedtime very low dose cyclobenzaprine on symptoms and sleep physiology in patients with fibromyalgia syndrome: a double-blind randomized placebo-controlled study. *J Rheumatol.*, 38, 2653-2663.

National Academies of Sciences, E., & Medicine. (2017). *The health effects of cannabis and cannabinoids: The current state of evidence and recommendations for research*: National Academies Press.

Richardson, K., Mattishent, K., Loke, Y.K., Steel, N., Fox, C., Grossi, C. M., . . . Savva, G. M. (2019). History of Benzodiazepine Prescriptions and Risk of Dementia: Possible Bias Due to Prevalent Users and Covariate Measurement Timing in a Nested Case-Control Study. *Am J Epidemiol, 188*(7), 1228–1236. doi:https://academic.oup.com/aje/article/188/7/1228/5421030

Rizzi, M., Sarzi-Puttini, P., Atzeni, F., Capsoni, F., Andreoli, A., Pecis, M., Colombo, S., Carrabba, M., & Sergi, M. (2004). Cyclic alternating pattern: a new marker of sleep alteration in patients with fibromyalgia? *J Rheumatol*, 31, 1193-1199.

Roizenblatt, S., Moldofsky, H., Benedito-Silva, A.A., & Tufik, S. (2001). Alpha sleep characteristics in fibromyalgia. *Arthritis Rheum.*, 44, 222-230.

Waters, K. (2021). Review of the Efficacy and Safety of Lemborexant, a Dual Receptor Orexin Antagonist (DORA), in the Treatment of Adults With Insomnia Disorder. *Annals of Pharmacotherapy*, 10600280211008492. doi:https://dx.doi.org/10.1177/10600280211008492

Session 3

Activity, Pacing, and the Autonomic Nervous System

Walk a Mile in My Shoe

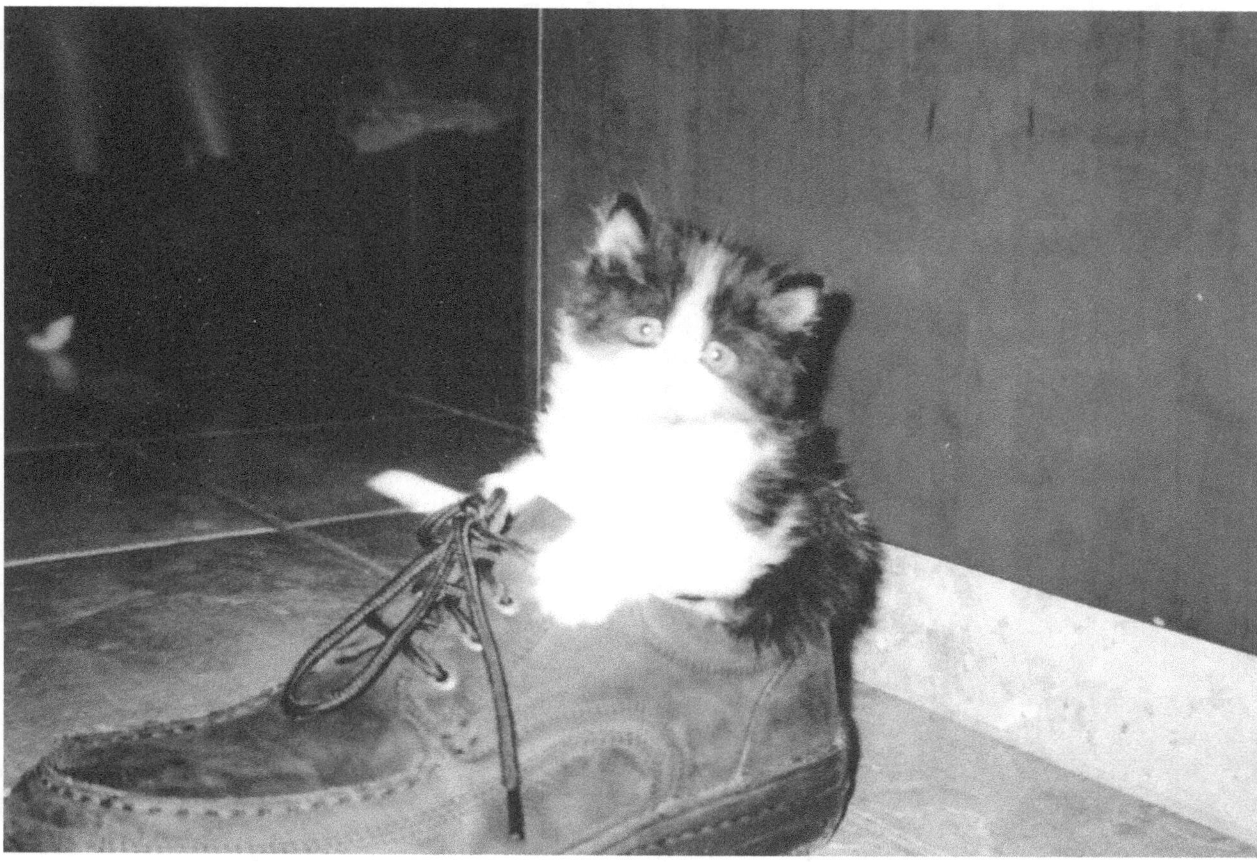

Inez & Rachel Stone of Cold Lake, AB

Session 3

Activity, Pacing, and the Autonomic Nervous System

Objectives

- To increase knowledge about activity and exercise in ME/CFS and FM.
- To use pacing and symptom monitoring to help you function at the maximum possible level for your health status.
- To find a sustainable balance between rest and activity.
- To understand the purpose of the autonomic nervous system.
- To understand the symptoms of autonomic dysfunction.
- To understand the treatment strategies for autonomic dysfunction.

There is limited reference to Multiple Chemical Sensitivity (MCS) in the first part of this session because people with MCS, in the absence of ME/CFS or FM, can usually exercise vigorously if they are not exposed to chemical triggers.

Does Exercise Improve ME/CFS?

Several well-publicized studies have reported that graded exercise therapy (GET) leads to improved energy and quality of life in patients with ME/CFS (Edmonds et al., 2004; White et al., 2011). While the studies showing improvement are frequently quoted—especially by insurance companies trying to get people back to work—several limitations in their methodology need to be considered.

- No published exercise study involving ME/CFS or FM has shown improvement in objective measures, such as a sustained increase in fitness or ability to return to work (or life roles) on a sustainable basis.
- Most of the studies reporting benefits from exercise in ME/CFS have used criteria such as the Oxford criteria that require very few symptoms for inclusion (e.g., fatigue and decreased function). These

non-specific criteria mean that, in addition to subjects with ME/CFS, subjects with depression or other conditions associated with fatigue are also 'erroneously' (if the purpose of the study is to look at what helps ME/CFS) included. Mood in depression is known to improve with regular exercise, so inclusion of depressed participants will make the results look better.

- Studies using the Fukuda or Canadian Consensus Criteria (recommended) have shown poorer outcomes. These are the two criteria for ME/CFS included in Session 1.

Contrasting with the well-publicized studies about the benefits of exercise in ME/CFS is a study from Belgium following real patients rather than research subjects. This multi-centre study, of over 1000 patients in 5 university clinics in Belgium, is the largest study published to date. The results showed that graded exercise helped more people feel better than worse as reported using self-report questionnaires (Stordeur et al., 2008). There was no improvement on tests of cardiovascular fitness.

- At the beginning of the study, the average participant worked at paid employment an average of 18.3% of a full-time (38 hours/ week) load. After the study, this dropped to 14.9%.
- Although people reported feeling better, this improvement did not allow them to work more (an objective measure of change). An important note about the Belgian study is that it is the only study to date with subjects who were "real patients." By this, I mean people who were referred by their physicians to the study clinics for treatment and were not rejected if they had other conditions or were using medications.

Lack of benefit from graded exercise therapy was replicated in a study by Jason and colleagues of non-drug treatments, including cognitive therapy, cognitive behavior therapy (including graded exercise), anaerobic exercise, and relaxation (Jason et al., 2007). For the 25 variables measured in this study, significant change occurred for 28%, 20%, 16%, and 12% of the variables for the cognitive, cognitive behavior therapy, anaerobic activity, and relaxation variables, respectively. The participants who did the cognitive therapies had the best results; however, most participants continued to meet diagnosable criteria for ME/CFS following the treatment trial.

People with post-exertional malaise who attempt to increase exercise/activity rarely realize the improvements reported in published studies. In fact, most people with ME/CFS report feeling worse. In a recent study of reported outcomes by 3925 patients, graded exercise has the lowest endorsement of any of the 150 treatments evaluated (Eckey et al., 2025). This worsening of symptoms is especially true if patients are not able to control the amount of exercise and the rate of increase. A publication notes that information on adverse effects is sparse in the studies reporting benefits of exercise in ME/CFS (Kindlon, 2011). How can we explain the difference between the reported research and real life?

Post-Exertional Malaise

It has become clear that the symptom of post-exertional malaise (PEM) underlies exercise intolerance. Patients often refer to PEM as a *crash* because the ability to function often comes to a sudden halt, unpredictably and without one's consent. Both the onset and the duration of PEM are variable and unpredictable. The unpredictability is especially problematic because it makes it hard to plan activities such as socializing or work. Sometimes one can manage a particular activity, and at other times not. Even the most careful pacing (as described below) can be insufficient to predictably complete planned activities unscathed by PEM.

By definition, recovery from a PEM crash takes more than 24 hours. Because of the duration of PEM, people with this disabling symptom cannot sustain the amount of activity that led to the crash on a repeated basis. This results in a decrease in the ability to function (Carruthers et al., 2003). In some cases, it takes days or even weeks to recover to baseline, and, sometimes, if the crash is very severe, recovery can be indefinite (Chu, Valencia, Garvert, & Montoya, 2018).

PEM can be triggered by relatively minor physical, cognitive or emotional activities—typically activities that were completed with ease prior to becoming ill. Sometimes PEM develops or is worsened due to external circumstances such as stressors or infection. Anything that increases the need for more cellular energy than one has available can cause PEM in an individual with ME, CFS or long COVID.

The research suggests that PEM is related to decreased energy metabolism in ME and long COVID (Appelman et al., 2024; Germain et al., 2022; Hoel et al., 2021; Yamano, Watanabe, & Kataoka, 2021). If this energy hypothesis is correct, it means that the mitochondria of people with ME/CFS are downregulated and, try as they may, they cannot push beyond this limitation.

Measuring Post-Exertional Malaise (PEM)

PEM is not just a theoretical construct. It can now be measured objectively. The cardiopulmonary exercise test (CPET) is the gold standard for measuring fitness and functional capacity. The amount of oxygen being used (VO2) is an objective measure of fitness. Patients with ME and CFS often show decreases in peak oxygen use (VO2 peak) and oxygen use at the anaerobic threshold (VAT), but this is inconsistent.

An argument has also been made that lower exercise capacity could be due to deconditioning, especially in people who have been ill for many years. With a single test, it is not possible to discount this interpretation. Many patients have been mistakenly told to exercise more based on this finding.

Staci Stephens, Mark Van Ness and their team at the Workwell Foundation (www.workwellfoundation.org/)

have developed a protocol that differentiates people with ME, CFS and long COVID from people who are out of shape. Their two-day CPET compares the values on the first and second consecutive days of identical testing. In healthy individuals, as well as in those with decreased capacity due to heart and lung disease, it is the norm for peak exercise capacity to be within a range of 8% on repeated tests. A decrease greater than 8% in oxygen use or work accomplished on Day 2 of the two-day protocol is an abnormal finding not found in other disease states or people who are deconditioned (Larson, 2018). It may be an objective measure of post-exertional malaise (Stevens, Snell, Stevens, Keller, & VanNess, 2018).

What makes this test especially useful is that it is possible to measure objectively whether an individual makes a maximal effort. If the scores show evidence of maximal effort on both days and the patient's capacity to do work (on the exercise bicycle) is lower on the second day, then the decreased work represents a failure to recover from the exercise the day before.

The Evolution of Guidelines on Activity Management in ME & CFS

To some, a discussion of graded exercise therapy may seem old news. However, sadly, in some jurisdictions, patients are still being forced into rehab programs based on exercise therapy and then are losing their disability support benefits when they are unable to continue or progress. Although we yearn for the day when this discussion is no longer needed, we are not there quite yet.

Serious concerns about the research on graded exercise therapy have come to light, in particular about the U.K. PACE trial. PACE was the largest controlled study to date to assess the impact of graded exercise therapy (GET) and cognitive behavioral therapy (CBT). Reports of very positive results were picked up in the media worldwide. However, a careful review of the methods used puts the results in question (Marks, 2017; Matthees, 2016).

In response to a request by patient advocates, a British court ordered the release of raw anonymized data to an independent statistician. The reanalysis drew very different conclusions than the study authors. In the independent review, there was no significant difference between the CBT (7% recovered) and GET (4% recovered) groups and the control group (3% recovered) (Wilshire, 2016).

Subsequent to this reanalysis and advocacy by patient groups, many important organisations changed their guidance.

- The Agency for Health Research and Quality (AHRQ) in the United States (https://www.ahrq.gov/) published a report in 2015 stating that there might be some benefits for some patients using cognitive behavioral therapy and graded exercise therapy. With the reanalysis of the PACE trial, the AHRQ published an addendum to its initial report (Smith et al., 2016), concluding there is insufficient evidence of benefit for either graded exercise therapy or cognitive behavior therapy in ME when subjects meeting the Oxford criteria were omitted.

- In July 2017, the U.S. Centers for Disease Control and Prevention (CDC) removed mention of CBT and GET therapies from its web page and renamed the condition ME/CFS rather than CFS (https://www.cdc.gov/me-cfs/index.html).
- In 2021, the National Institute for Health and Care Excellence (NICE) in the U.K. updated its guidelines for diagnosis and management of ME/CFS (National Institute for Health and Care Excellence, 2021). The institute now recommends pacing guided by the patient and the patient's response to various activities, i.e., listening to the body. They specifically recommend against fixed incremental increases in activity, as is used in GET. They recommend CBT as an aid in symptom management, but stress that it is not a curative treatment for ME/CFS.

There is now widespread agreement that ME and CFS are serious biomedical conditions with significant energy and activity limitations, not caused by deconditioning and that these limitations must be respected day to day to optimize function. Hopefully, we can now move on and focus on pacing as the primary management strategy while awaiting clinical trials of biomedical strategies to increase mitochondrial function.

Exercise Therapy for Fibromyalgia

The Fibromyalgia literature supports the effectiveness of both moderate aerobic exercise and weight training (Brosseau et al, 2008a; Brosseau et al, 2008b). Studies report improvements in subjective measures of mood, quality of life, and pain, with 8- 10-week activity programs. In the Brosseau reviews, completed at the University of Ottawa, improvement was defined as greater than 15% change between pre- and post-exercise program functioning.

Most of the improvements are statistically significant, meaning that the probability they could have occurred by chance is very small. But few of the improvements are clinically significant. This means that the participants felt better, but there was no real change to their daily lives. Not all studies showed positive change, and most were small studies.

None of the studies measured participants' ability to return (with treatment) to previously enjoyed activities or work. Nevertheless, in real life, it seems that in keeping with the research, patients with FM do tolerate and benefit from suitable exercise programs.

It is true, however, that **if people don't remain active, over time they will become less fit, lose muscle mass, and become less mobile**. People who are deconditioned are more liable to falls and accidents because of a decrease in balance and slower reflexes. Therefore, it is critical for people with ME/CFS and FM to remain active enough to forestall these adverse consequences while at the same time not overdoing it and making themselves worse. Finding the right balance is akin to walking a tightrope. I am not focusing on MCS here since most of these patients are able to remain active.

The objective of this session is to provide information and ideas to help you find the right balance for you. To understand why some of the recommendations about exercise are being made, it is important to have a **basic** understanding of exercise physiology. You don't need to know all the details to appreciate how healthy bodies react with exercise and how people with ME/CFS and FM differ from the norm.

Aerobic and Anaerobic Exercise Physiology

In healthy people, **resting heart rate (HR) is 60 - 72 beats per minute (bpm).** As a person exercises, heart rate and blood pressure gradually rise. The **aerobic window** is the heart rate range within which energy is generated from oxygen and glucose. In this range, exercise can be sustained for a long time, even hours, in fit individuals. Exercising in this range improves fitness and burns calories. The aerobic window is a function of age. The aerobic window ranges between 60 - 80% of the age-adjusted maximum heart rate. To calculate the age-adjusted maximum heart rate, subtract your age from 220. For a fifty-year-old person, the age-adjusted maximum heart rate (220 – 50) is 170. The aerobic window is 60 to 80% of this (170 x 0.6 - 170 x 0.8) or approximately 102 – 136 bpm.

For a healthy person with a resting heart rate of 60 beats per minute and an aerobic window of up to 140 bpm, there is a lot of room (140 - 60 = 80 bpm) to *train*. Training refers to the ability to increase the intensity or duration of exercise over time as a result of consistent exertion and appropriate rest. With intensities above the upper limit of the aerobic heart rate window, the body begins to rely on anaerobic metabolism, the burning of glucose without oxygen. Anaerobic metabolism can only last for a short time and is associated with the buildup of lactic acid.

People with ME/CFS (especially those who are severely ill) are unable to benefit from exercise in the same way as healthy people. People with ME/CFS report an increase in many of their symptoms after exercise. And this exacerbation of symptoms lasts for more than 24 hours (see the Canadian Consensus Definition of ME/CFS in Session 1).

A study of genetic expression before and after exercise suggests a possible reason why this might be the case. The immune system (complement pathway) is triggered by exercise much more in people with ME/CFS than in controls, and doesn't return to normal after exercise (Light et al., 2009). The same patterns are **not** seen in patients with FM (in the absence of ME/CFS) or in patients with multiple sclerosis (Light et al., 2012).

Most patients with ME/CFS and FM have a high resting heart rate of > 80 bpm. The normal resting heart rate range is 60 - 72 bpm. Very fit people have an even lower heart rate, often 50 - 60 bpm. This increase is thought to be a sign of dysfunction of the autonomic nervous system (ANS), the part of the nervous system that controls all the involuntary functions (see more on this in the section on the ANS below).

A subset of people with ME/CFS has a decreased **aerobic threshold**. This means that they begin producing lactic acid at a heart rate as low as 110 bpm instead of 140 bpm or higher (Lund et al., 2003; Lane et al., 1998). The combination of a high resting heart rate and a lower aerobic threshold means that the potential aerobic training window is narrower. For people with a resting heart rate of over 100 bpm, the aerobic training window is nonexistent.

The most accurate way to measure the aerobic threshold is with a treadmill or bicycle exercise test. As a person exercises at increasingly more strenuous levels, heart rate and blood lactate are measured. When the blood lactate level starts increasing, this means that the body is using anaerobic metabolism. As a rough guide for those who haven't had an exercise test done, the aerobic/lactate threshold is approximately the heart rate at which a person is breathing too hard to talk easily.

One way to measure recovery from activity is by how quickly the heart rate returns to its baseline after resting. Athletes use the morning resting heart rate to plan their workouts for the day. If heart rate is fully recovered (i.e., as low as it was the day before), the workout can be more intense without ill effects. If heart rate has not recovered from the day before and remains higher than usual, activity should be moderated to allow the body to recover. Continued high activity without full heart rate recovery leads to overtraining syndrome. Overtraining is associated with decreased performance at the same or increased effort. For athletes, this is often experienced as fatigue. Overtraining syndrome in athletes shares many characteristics in common with ME/CFS.

Joan's Activity Log

When reading this section, have Joan's Activity Chart (pg. 2-20) and her energy ratings (pg. 2-21, and your own charting to refer to. Look for similarities between your chart(s) and Joan's. Then use these and the discussion that follows to evaluate whether you could make changes to your own activity pattern.

You can see from Joan's chart that she has a fairly regular daily routine. She gets up between 8:00 am and 9:30 am. It takes her a couple of hours to get up, shower if needed, get dressed, and eat. Then, if she is not working, she takes her dog for a short walk in the neighbourhood. She walks slowly because of her sore ankle.

In the middle of the day, Joan does most of her *necessary tasks,* such as shopping, appointments, cleaning, and cooking. This is when her physical and mental energy are at their peak. During this charting period, she had a couple of social activities during the week, including a family Boxing Day celebration and a New Year's Eve party with a friend.

Some days, Joan takes a rest during the day and other days she doesn't, depending on her fatigue level and the time she has available. You can see that most evenings she is very tired, spending time on the couch reading, watching TV, or resting with the dog. She rarely has the energy to go out in the evening, something she used to enjoy, as that is when her friends are available to spend time. Unfortunately for Joan, most nights her energy level falls by 7 - 8 pm to the "couch potato" level. Although she is very tired, she doesn't go to bed early since, from experience, she knows she won't sleep before 11 pm. Even though exhausted, with energy levels of between 30 and 40%, it still takes her over an hour to fall asleep most nights.

Comparing Joan's functional capacity at the start and end of each day, you can see that there is a significant drop between morning and evening. This is shown by the downwards arrows on the Sleep Chart at the end of Session 2. This means that Joan is functioning outside her individual *energy envelope* and is running a daily energy debt. Just as with money, one can run a debt for a while, but over time, the interest piles up, and one gets into trouble. Joan is at risk of a crash if additional responsibilities, stressors, or sleep disruption were to occur. We'll talk about the energy envelope later in this session and how to avoid the push/crash cycle.

What does your activity chart look like? Are you running an energy debt, too?

It may be helpful for Joan to try taking a purposeful rest in the middle of the day to see if this provides her with a bit better energy at the end of the day and to avoid going into an energy debt. A purposeful rest is very different than "couch time." Purposeful resting/napping means lying down with eyes and ears closed, either resting or meditating. It does NOT include watching TV, reading, or listening to music, unless the music is very relaxing. I learned about purposeful napping from Dr. Alison Bested when she talked in Calgary in 2008.

Since then, many patients have told me that they are surprised how well it works. Many of us think we have to actually sleep to feel better; however, some people benefit from purposeful naps. We don't know exactly why purposeful resting is helpful. It may be that the horizontal position ensures better blood flow to the brain. And the relaxation part of the rest may help the body learn and remember how to calm down and relax, as does formal meditation. Some patients report better sleep at night when they have purposefully rested during the day.

Another pacing strategy is to break up activities into shorter intervals. While cooking, doing laundry, or cleaning, this would entail working for only 10 - 20 minutes, then taking a similar length break and coming back to the activity. At the moment, Joan appears to tackle most tasks in one lump rather than splitting them up. Most people find that tackling a task and finishing it is gratifying, and they don't want to split it up. However, it may be that splitting a task such as cooking (that requires standing) into short periods will enable you to cook more healthy food than if you give up cooking because it is too exhausting.

Joan seems to have slept longer on the days after she took a purposeful rest, but she will need to continue monitoring to see if this pattern continues. This chart (without the sleep quality data) does not show whether the sleep was restorative, merely how long she slept. To evaluate the restorativeness of sleep, you need to use the Sleep Chart or add an extra row to the Activity Log.

Interpretation of Sleep Charts is made more complicated by the possibility that you could have a delayed or cumulative response to either activity or rest (or food or stress, etc.). This makes it harder to determine the connection between activity and symptoms. In many people, the effects of stressors are cumulative and may not hit until a few days or even weeks after ongoing exposure to a new activity, food, scent, or a combination of events or exposures.

How to Exercise Safely and Effectively

People with ME/CFS, FM and MCS want to be able to do the activities they enjoy without exacerbating their symptoms. There are now several published papers suggesting how to do this (Jones & Clark, 2002; Nijs et al., 2008; Jason et al., 2008). None of the approaches in these papers, or recommended by me in this manual, utilizes the forced graded exercise approach (known as Graded Exercise Therapy or GET). Although reported to be of use in a few prominent papers, my experience is that a forced increase in activity of any kind, not paying attention to symptom changes, often results in relapse.

This section focuses on strategies for stabilizing and increasing activity level and fitness using pacing as a primary strategy and tools such as HR, Heart Rate Variability, and exercise testing as additional tools.

General Guidelines

Maintaining and increasing fitness is a worthwhile goal. However, intentional exercise should not be undertaken at the cost of daily functioning. Exercise makes most people feel better psychologically and increases mood. Although there are overlaps in the symptom profiles of people with ME/CFS and FM, response to exercise is one way in which the two groups differ. If your only diagnosis is MCS and you do not have activity limitations, then this section does not apply to you. Consider yourself lucky and move on to the section on the Autonomic Nervous System later in this session.

- Patients with either ME/CFS or FM who have severe to extreme illness severity (**average daily energy levels below 50%**), and those with additional blood pressure and infectious symptoms, rarely benefit from exercise over and above the amount needed for daily function. Graded exercise (not forced) may still be helpful to increase tolerance of activities of daily living. However, for the severely ill, activity should be integrated into the daily routine rather than being added on top as intentional exercise. Examples of daily routines that are *activities* for moderately to severely ill patients include standing to prepare food, doing laundry, going up and down stairs, light housework, talking on the phone, and working on the computer. Remember that mental activity uses energy and can be just as exhausting as physical activity.
- Patients with ME/CFS or FM who have an **average daily energy level between 50 and 80%** may exercise but should keep the heart rate below their individual aerobic/lactate threshold. As noted earlier, a rough guide for those who haven't had an exercise test done, the aerobic/lactate threshold is approximately the heart rate at which a person is breathing too hard to talk easily. Details of the lactate test are discussed later in this session.
- Patients with ME/CFS or FM with an average daily **energy level above 80%** may experiment with more strenuous exercise, increasing the heart rate into the normal aerobic exercise range for their age.

Working on Attitudes About Exercise

It is a widely held belief that exercise is "good for people," and people who do not exercise are not doing all they can to help themselves. Most people have grown up with these beliefs, and they are frequently heard from the mouths of physicians and family members. In fact, many people with ME/CFS and FM had these attitudes towards others before becoming ill. It is difficult to consider that these assumptions may not be true for everyone. Being physically fit is often an integral part of self-image, and to refrain from exercising the way a person did before becoming ill requires a huge psychological adjustment.

Recovery from ME/CFS and FM requires a new understanding of the relationship between energy and health, one that respects your body's limits rather than trying to push through them. There is a small group of patients who fear that any activity will set them back and who have become activity-avoidant. Listening to the body and using objective tools such as exercise testing and heart rate monitoring lessens the chance that one will go too far wrong, either in the direction of too much or too little activity.

Finding Your Energy Envelope

- The energy envelope refers to the **finite** amount of energy one has available to use in a day. Note that in healthy people, energy is **not** considered finite. It can be increased by a healthy diet, adequate sleep, and training. In people with ME/CFS, and to a lesser extent FM, the envelope seems limited.

- The Adapted Karnofsky Rating Scale will help you determine your current energy level. You have already used this scale to fill in the *Sleep Chart* after Session 1 and to complete the Activity Log after Session 2.
- Estimate your energy level each morning using this scale and mark that level on your Sleep Chart or Activity Log.
- Record your energy level again at the end of the day. Notice if there is a difference between your energy at the beginning and end of each day. By drawing an arrow on the graph portion of the Sleep Chart between the morning and afternoon scores, you create a visual record of whether you are gaining or losing energy each day. For example, if you started the day at 60% energy but by the end of the day couldn't get off the couch (< 30%), this would be a decrease of 30% shown by a downward arrow reaching from 60% to 30%.
- If your chart is filled with *downward arrows* (i.e., you are far more tired at the end of the day than at the beginning), then you are consistently exceeding your energy envelope. To improve your health, you must learn to live within your energy means.

Staying Within Your Energy Envelope

If you consistently have downward arrows on your Sleep Chart or Activity Log, you are operating outside your energy envelope, and your health is less likely to improve than if you stay within the envelope. Leonard Jason's research has shown that people who stay within their energy envelope have the ability to increase their activity levels over time (Jason et al., 2009).

People functioning within their envelopes report less fatigue than people who consistently overspend on their energy account. This could be summarized as "pay now or pay later." If you exceed your energy limit now, you will pay later by failing to recover over the long term. If you hold back and pace better now, you may be able to recover over the long term and enjoy better, stable energy in the future.

Therefore, the **first goal of activity management** for patients with ME/CFS and FM is to use only as much energy as you have each day. You want to end each day with as much energy as you started with and minimize downward energy arrows. Once average daily energy is stable, sustainable, and predictable, you can experiment with adding activity in a graduated manner.

A Helpful Metaphor

- **Treat energy like money**. Unlike healthy people who restore energy throughout the day with rest and food, and each night with sleep, you have a finite amount of energy to spend each day. You choose whether to stay within your energy budget or to overspend.

- Just like with a line of credit or a credit card, you can overspend for special occasions. However, you will accumulate a debt that must be repaid. If you overspend consistently, you will have to pay back the accumulated debt **with interest**.
- Maintaining a high financial or energy debt is both psychologically and physically stressful. It leaves you with no reserve for the inevitable rainy day.
- If you overspend your exercise account either in intensity, frequency, or duration, your energy will decrease over time because you will be using some of your energy each day to pay off your energy debt. Just as with a national debt, if you spend too much of your daily resources paying off past debt, you won't have energy to spend on things that arise in the future.
- Like a credit counsellor, I advise all patients to pay off their energy debts and commit to living "debt-free."
- If you do less activity than your body needs, you will feel stiff and lethargic.
- If you pace yourself correctly, your energy and exercise capacity will stabilize and slowly increase—not because you have exercised but because you have listened to your body and are being fiscally responsible with respect to energy.

Signs of Overspending

- If you feel anxious or "hyper" after any activity, this may be because you overdid it and triggered the production of **adrenaline**. In this metaphor, energy is money; adrenaline is your credit card. You can use it when you don't have money in the bank to pay, and it will buy you time. Adrenaline, like caffeine, leaves you ready for action and will make relaxation and sleep more difficult.
- The tell-tale sign of increased adrenaline levels is increased heart rate. Taking your heart rate at the beginning and end of each day is another way to estimate if you are staying within your energy envelope or are using your adrenaline credit card. If your heart rate is similar at the end of the day to what it was at the beginning, you are using adrenaline responsibly.
- Heart rate (HR) increases with activity and returns to resting level when the body has recovered. In healthy people, this occurs within 24 hours for daily activities (it takes longer to recover from very high activity levels like running a marathon).
- By taking your heart rate each morning before getting out of bed, you can see if you have recovered from the previous day. A higher-than-normal heart rate means that you have **not** recovered. I'll talk later about the Tools of the Trade, with the heart rate monitor being one option.

Attempting Increased Activity

- You should only attempt increases in activity after energy stabilization has occurred.
- Start with an easily obtainable activity goal, one just slightly above what you currently tolerate (based on stable, consistent daily energy levels).
- An example of a concrete activity goal is walking for 10 minutes at a heart rate (HR) maximum of 110 bpm on alternate days.

I am frequently asked how to pick a starting point for exercise intensity.

- If you haven't been able to move much, you should start at approximately 55 –65% of predicted age-adjusted maximal heart rate.
- If you are not very deconditioned, but have not yet started to attempt graded exercise, pick the 65% level – you can always increase.
- For a 50-year-old individual, the calculation is (220 – age) X 0.55 = 93 bpm; (220 – age) X 0.65 = 110bpm, so that the range would be between 93 and 110 bpm. Note that this isn't a very high HR and may not give you much room to play with. Some people fall into despair after purchasing their HR monitor and realize how much they have been "overdoing" it.

An alternative (and more hopeful) perspective is that at least now you have an accurate way to measure your energy envelope! Just as people with diabetes use blood sugar levels to monitor their progress, some patients with ME/CFS and FM can use HR. NOTE: Not all patients with ME/CFS and FM have an elevated or reactive heart rate. If your HR is always quite low (i.e., below 65bpm) and doesn't go up very much even with exercise, HR monitoring may not be as useful a tool for you. It doesn't mean that your system is functioning better, just differently.

Remember that Leonard Jason's work shows that if you function consistently within your energy envelope, it will expand over time. If you get frustrated and try to push through, you are likely to suffer a setback. People who are in better condition and are less ill can start their exercise at a higher heart rate. You will have to experiment to see what exercise intensity you can keep up for a couple of weeks.

- Maintain this new activity level for 2 weeks and chart your pre- and post-activity energy levels.

In this manual, we will be moving on to charting stressful events and then discussing *Coping* over the next 2 weeks. If you are really struggling to find your energy envelope, consider continuing your focus on this session before moving on. If you feel you can chart more than one thing at a time, then forge ahead.

- Your body will let you know when you have it "right" by responding with consistent energy over the day and then from one day to the next.

- After maintaining an activity goal for 1 month and noticing a stable or improved energy level, the activity goal may be increased by up to 10% (e.g., if you are at 10 minutes, then try 11 minutes).
- If at any point symptoms increase daily, energy decreases or becomes less stable, or morning or evening heart rates begin to increase, activity goals should be decreased until restabilization occurs.
- If your energy level is temporarily affected by factors such as illness, injury, lack of sleep, or psychological stress, a temporary decrease in activity may help you recover faster.

Pacing Tips by Bruce Campbell

Bruce Campbell is a psychologist who has ME/CFS. He used his knowledge and expertise to develop a self-management program, which allowed him to recover considerably. He founded a website offering the program he developed through moderated internet discussion groups. He has written a manual to accompany the course. His manual utilizes many of the same concepts as this manual and will complement nicely what you learn here. A benefit of the https://cfsselfhelp.org/ course is that you will be able to interact with others learning the same skills and can compare notes with others in the virtual group. Here are some of Dr. Campbell's pacing tips:

- Routine: Make a schedule to minimize unexpected activities that drain energy.
- Rest: In between activities, some people say even 5 minutes of horizontal rest makes a difference. I've already touched a bit on this when I talked about purposeful resting.
- Short Activity Periods: Breaking activities into short periods of 15 – 30 minutes will allow you to accomplish more than doing the entire activity at once and then crashing.
- Task Switching: Switching between tasks that use different parts of the brain or body to give other parts of the body a rest.
- Prioritizing: Don't keep a list of a kazillion (my wording, not his) tasks to do. Figure out which tasks are really critical and use your energy to do these well.
- Honouring Time of Day: Schedule important tasks when you have the most energy.
- Pacing While Driving: Take breaks while driving to stop, stretch, and drink, and arrive refreshed and calm rather than exhausted and frazzled.

Tools of the Trade

As mentioned above, a heart rate (HR) monitor is, in my opinion, an essential tool for those who are working to find and stay within their energy envelope. Patients with MCS may also benefit from using an HR monitor for different reasons. Increased HR is a common reaction to chemical exposure in patients with MCS. If you are frequently impacted and/or have a poor sense of smell, using an HR monitor is a way to objectively measure the impact of chemical exposures. Some patients with MCS don't have HR reactions to chemicals. So, it's best to try borrowing a monitor from a friend or local retailer and using it for a couple of weeks to see if you think it will be helpful. Most sports enthusiasts, especially runners, use HR monitors to help them plan and monitor their workouts. Like you, they don't want to develop symptoms from overtraining.

Heart Rate (HR) Monitor

An HR monitor consists of a transmitter that picks up and transmits your heartbeat, now most commonly in the form of a watch or ring. The best type of monitor to buy is one with audible alarms, which will go off when you are out of range. If, for example, you are trying to stay under your aerobic threshold while doing daily activities, you can set the monitor to beep if you exceed this number. The beeping allows you to go about your day without having to look at the watch.

You could use an HR monitor as described above to alert you when you are exceeding a particular HR. However, the monitor can also help you figure out what your maximal heart rate for daily activities should be. If you wear the monitor daily and glance at it from time to time, you will become familiar with your HR range. Notice if this range differs on days when you feel well at the end of the day and sleep well, compared with days when you end the day crashed on the couch. By doing this, you may be able to notice within which HR range you function best. Other ways to use an HR monitor include

- Charting your heart rate during the day (especially at times when you feel especially good or bad) to see if heart rate is an accurate indicator for you.
- Noting the heart rate at which you begin to feel any of pain, fatigue, lightheadedness, abdominal cramps, or need to urinate. If you charted your heart rate as suggested in the first bullet, note if you suffer fatigue the next day. If you have had any of the consequences listed (pain, fatigue, etc. or delayed fatigue), experiment with keeping your heart rate below this number for several days in a row. Does this affect your health?
- Noticing how the same activity may be associated with different heart rates and different body reactions from one day to the next. Your body is constantly changing in reaction to internal and external conditions.
- If your heart rate is especially high or labile (changes easily), you may wish to chart your morning and evening heart rate on your Sleep Chart. As your heart rate stabilizes, you will know you are on the right track.

Pedometer

A pedometer measures the number of steps you take per day. It is a small, light instrument that is worn hooked onto a belt or waistband. Healthy people are told to aim for 10,000 steps per day. This is roughly equivalent to walking 10 km throughout a day, including walking around the house, walking to do errands, etc. Here are some ways to use a pedometer:

- Record your daily steps every day for two weeks on your Sleep Chart. You can make a new column or use one of the existing columns to record this. Then look at the patterns to determine what your optimal *step count per day* is, in order to maintain energy.
- For most people with ME/CFS and FM, too many steps will lead to a decline in energy, and too few will lead to stiffness and pain. This is different from what occurs in healthy people.
- Your optimal *steps per day* will vary from a good day to a bad day.
- Maintain a step/day level which minimizes symptoms over a period of 2 -3 months. This will stabilize energy and health and allow you to start making progress.
- Though not as helpful as a heart rate monitor, the pedometer is cheaper and easier to use.

What about Cognitive Activity?

I also get asked frequently why there is no chapter on cognition. The brain needs energy just like the body. In people with PEM, there is insufficient energy, and this may be a cause of the common symptom of brain fog. Just as pacing will help improve physical function, as a general rule, if you are able to keep your daily energy level steady for several months, your cognition will begin to improve. Improvement in cognition generally lags several months behind improvement in physical function and other symptoms. So don't get discouraged.

It is not clear yet whether doing brain exercise (e.g., paper or computerized cognitive challenges) will improve cognitive function in ME/CFS, FM and MCS. Currently, there are no studies that look at this. It is different treating the cognitive problems in ME/CFS, FM and MCS than helping a person recover from a stroke. The damage from a stroke is presumably finished, whereas the forces causing cognitive problems in ME/CFS, FM and MCS are ongoing.

Remember that cognitive exercise can be just as exhausting as physical exercise for patients with ME/CFS, FM and MCS. Therefore, if you undertake a program of brain exercise, you should follow the same pacing strategies that you follow when undertaking physical exercise.

The Autonomic Nervous System

The autonomic nervous system (ANS) controls most of the involuntary functions of the body, including blood pressure, breathing, bowel and bladder function, sweating, sexual function, and more. The ANS is important for homeostasis—the body's ability to react to and adjust to external and internal changes. Examples include adjusting to standing, running, eating, or urinating. Autonomic nervous system dysfunction is common among people with ME/CFS, FM and MCS.

Discussion of the autonomic nervous system is included here since it strongly impacts HR and the ability to exercise. Most people with ANS dysfunction will have awareness of having some of the symptoms listed below. These symptoms reflect the body's inability to respond as needed to changes in environment and activity, including the specific challenge of standing upright. Note that there are many other causes of the symptoms below. The symptoms that are the most specific to ANS are marked with an asterisk.

- ☐ Dizziness *
- ☐ Palpitations*
- ☐ Blurred vision
- ☐ Clamminess
- ☐ Anxiety
- ☐ Fatigue
- ☐ Headache
- ☐ Symptoms relieved by lying down*
- ☐ Able to stand in line < 20 minutes*
- ☐ Symptoms worsen after moderately heavy meals
- ☐ Irritable Bowel symptoms
- ☐ Irritable Bladder symptoms
- ☐ Too much or too little sweating
- ☐ Sexual symptoms (erectile dysfunction and low libido)
- ☐ Light-headedness*
- ☐ Exercise intolerance
- ☐ Chest discomfort
- ☐ Lower limb swelling
- ☐ Flushing
- ☐ Nausea
- ☐ Loss of consciousness*
- ☐ Shortness of breath
- ☐ Weakness

The ANS is especially critical for maintaining blood flow to the brain. The brain requires a constant supply of blood, carrying oxygen and nutrients to function. If the brain does not get enough nutrition, symptoms such as dizziness, weakness, nausea, muscle pain, and *brain fog* develop within seconds.

Single-photon emission computed tomography (SPECT) brain blood flow studies have confirmed that there is insufficient blood flow to several parts of the brain in persons with ME/CFS and MCS (Ichise et al., 1992). Lack of adequate blood flow to the brain and other organs while standing causes symptoms of orthostatic intolerance (Streeten & Bell, 1998). This lack of blood flow to critical organs is due both to not having enough blood and to the tendency of the blood to leak out of the blood vessels and into the tissues (Stewart & Weldon, 2000).

Orthostatic intolerance (OI) is the development of symptoms when sitting or standing upright. It is a clinical syndrome common (if not universal) in people with autonomic nervous system dysfunction and common in people with ME/CFS (Newton et al., 2007). People with FM and MCS are not as routinely affected by orthostatic intolerance. Chronic orthostatic intolerance is a disabling condition that can severely affect quality of life (Furlan et al., 1998; Benrud-Larson et al., 2002). Interestingly, OI is associated with severe fatigue!

Two diagnostic categories may be found in people complaining of orthostatic intolerance: neurally mediated hypotension (NMH) and postural orthostatic tachycardia Syndrome (POTS).

In **neurally mediated hypotension** (NMH), the nerve signals that compensate for the change in position (i.e., lying to standing) malfunction. As a result, the decrease in blood pressure while standing lasts longer and is more severe than it should be. To avoid injury due to lack of oxygen, the brain tells the body to lie down quickly (it is easier to pump blood horizontally than vertically). This is experienced as sudden dizziness or fainting upon standing.

Although NMH can be diagnosed clinically (a person falls over when s/he tries to stand), a formal diagnosis requires a Tilt Table Test. In this test, a patient is strapped to a table and heart rate and blood pressure monitors are put on. The table is slowly tilted to a 70-degree head-up position, and HR and BP are monitored. In NMH, the BP will drop, and the patient will report dizziness and then pass out.

In **postural orthostatic tachycardia syndrome** (POTS), the blood pressure with standing is relatively normal, but the heart rate speeds up to try to pump blood more quickly to the organs. If this compensation is insufficient, the person feels dizzy, tired, weak, nauseous, AND has a rapid pounding heartbeat. The formal diagnosis is made by noting an increase in HR of 28 beats per minute or to a level of more than 110 beats per minute. If the BP falls by more than 20/10 or the difference between the higher and lower BP numbers falls to less than 18mm Hg (pulse pressure), a diagnosis can also be made. There is more about Blood Pressure in the next section, under Blood Pressure Monitoring.

Diagnosing Autonomic Dysfunction

As already noted, the autonomic nervous system controls many aspects of the body's function. Heart rate and blood pressure offer a valuable, non-invasive window into the ANS.

The clinicians at the Bateman Horne Center have developed a test easily done at home or in a doctor's office to identify autonomic dysfunction (Vernon et al., 2022). Full instructions can be found at https://batemanhornecenter.org/nasa-10-minute-lean-test-2/.

NASA Lean Test

Preparation

- Rest lying down for at least 10 minutes to establish baseline vitals.
- Record heart rate (HR) and blood pressure (BP) at the end of rest.

Positioning

- Stand upright with your back against a wall, heels 6–8 inches from the wall, and shoulders/buttocks touching the wall.
- This prevents muscle pumping from shifting weight and helps standardize the test.
- Rest your arms at your sides with feet flat and avoid movement or fidgeting.

Test Procedure

- Duration: 10 minutes (some protocols go up to 20 minutes if tolerated).
- Measure and record HR and BP at each minute. This requires a blood pressure cuff and an assistant who knows how to use it.
- Watch for symptoms: dizziness, palpitations, foggy brain, fatigue, nausea, pale complexion or chest pain.
- Watch for pooling of the blood in the feet, causing discoloration or swelling.

Postural orthostatic tachycardia syndrome (POTS): HR increase ≥30 bpm (≥40 bpm in adolescents) within 10 minutes, without significant BP drop.

Orthostatic hypotension: Systolic BP drop ≥20 mmHg or diastolic drop ≥10 mmHg within 3 minutes.

Neurally mediated hypotension/syncope: Delayed sudden BP and HR drop with symptoms.

Be aware that this test underdiagnoses. Sophisticated testing of blood flow to the head with Doppler ultrasound shows that some people have significantly decreased blood flow even when BP and heart rate are relatively stable (van Campen, Verheugt, Rowe, & Visser, 2020).

Treatment of Orthostatic Intolerance (OI)

We currently lack effective methods to treat the root causes of autonomic dysfunction. There are drugs to treat some specific symptoms (e.g., bowel or bladder spasm or to speed bowel transit time), but we have no treatment for whatever it is that makes the ANS not respond as it should. Some autonomic disorders are autoimmune diseases. That is, the body produces antibodies that damage the autonomic nerves or deplete the supply of necessary neurotransmitters. Some treatments are being tested to identify and remove the offending antibodies (Wirth & Scheibenbogen, 2020).

This section deals only with orthostatic intolerance, which, by now, you will know, is one of the manifestations of autonomic dysfunction. Some of the bowel symptoms common in ME/CFS, FM and MCS may also be related to autonomic dysfunction. Treatments for these symptoms will be covered in Session 5 in the section on irritable bowel syndrome.

Of course, before attempting any intervention such as changing your blood pressure or blood volume (the treatment of choice for OI), it is always a good idea to consult with your family physician. You might find, however, that physicians are relatively uninterested in helping you **increase** your blood pressure. In over 20 years of attending medical education seminars and conferences, I have never heard (outside the environmental medicine and ME/CFS circles) a single talk on the health consequences of low blood pressure. Patients with symptomatically low BP are often told their blood pressure is “excellent” and that they are at low risk for a heart attack or stroke. While this is true (about the risk of heart attack and stroke), low blood flow to the brain is associated with all the cognitive problems experienced daily by patients with ME/CFS, FM and MCS. Low blood pressure is not a benign condition. Normalizing BP can lead to a significant improvement in quality of life.

Conservative (non-drug) Treatment for Orthostatic Intolerance

The most successful treatments for OI are those that increase the amount of blood in the body (blood volume) and its distribution (blood pressure).

- Before trying any interventions for your blood pressure, you must acquire a blood pressure monitor and use it daily to ensure that you are moving closer to the normal range and are not overshooting.
- The first intervention is to stop doing the things that make the problem worse. For instance, you may need to stop avoiding salt. It is widely known that added salt “is bad” because it causes an increase in blood pressure and risk of heart attack and stroke. While that may be true for the majority of adults, it is NOT true for those patients with ME/CFS who have low blood pressure (Newton et al., 2009). So, after confirming that your BP is actually low, stop avoiding salt.

- Many patients with orthostatic intolerance, especially those who get swelling in the legs, report benefit from support hose. For support hose to work, they should be fitted by a professional and fit tightly enough to constrain the blood flow to the lower limbs. The same feature that makes them effective also makes them uncomfortable. Most medical supply stores will be able to direct you to such an individual, and larger stores may have someone on staff qualified to fit you. Support hose is especially helpful when standing for periods of time (e.g., shopping or attending social functions) and/or when taking a flight of more than a couple of hours in length.
- After support hose, the most commonly recommended treatment for orthostatic intolerance is to increase salt and water intake. For this purpose, use salt as a drug; take a measured amount regularly throughout the day, not just when you think of it. A common approach is to start with 1/4 teaspoon of sea salt or Kosher salt (i.e., without additives) and increase the dose to four times daily as needed. The section on Increasing Blood Volume in Session 9 contains more on this. When you increase salt intake, you will naturally become thirstier. Drink as indicated by your body. There is no need to drink more than 2 litres per day unless you are really thirsty. Drinking too much can cause health problems. Improvement may be noted in energy, cognitive function, and decreased urine output.
- Maintain adequate protein intake. Protein in the blood helps retain fluid in the blood vessels rather than it leaking into the tissues.
- Ensure that blood pressure/heart rate reactions are not due to food or chemical exposures. If they are, alter your diet and environment to minimize these reactions. Many people with MCS develop low blood pressure and a high heart rate when exposed to toxins.
- If you develop swelling when upright, keep your feet elevated to prevent swelling and use properly fitted support hose when upright for long periods of time.
- When standing, be sure to move regularly and flex the calf and leg muscles to keep blood from flowing back to the heart.
- Mild exercise generally improves orthostatic intolerance, but moderate to intense exercise in people with ME/CFS may worsen symptoms since the blood will be going to the muscles instead of other critical organs.

Medications for Orthostatic Intolerance

Fludrocortisone (Florinef®) is an artificial form of aldosterone, the hormone that instructs the kidneys to retain salt and water. Some patients don't respond to salt and water alone; they just urinate it out. This drug can prevent that and is a staple treatment for orthostatic intolerance. The usual dose is 0.1 mg in the morning. Some people with severe symptoms may need an additional 1/2 dose later in the day.

Midodrine® is a medication that increases vascular tone. This is helpful for people who have "floppy" small arteries. In patients who develop low blood pressure and lower extremity swelling, midodrine can improve symptoms.

Pyridostigmine bromide (Mestinon®) is a medication that blocks the breakdown of acetyl choline, the neurotransmitter that enables parasympathetic and muscular function. It increases parasympathetic tone and decreases heart rate. Pyridostigmine is generally well tolerated if used as directed and if the dose is increased slowly over 10 – 14 days.

If you get increased salivation or watering eyes, consider lowering the dose. Avoid in combination with beta blockers or if your heart rate is already below 60 beats/minute. Start at 30 mg once daily and work up as tolerated to 60 mg twice daily or the best dose to decrease symptoms and increase function.

If at any time while treating your low BP, you notice that your BP is getting too high, meet again with your physician to try to work out the problem. High blood pressure on a consistent basis increases the risk of heart attack and stroke and should be avoided.

For more on diagnosis and treatment of orthostatic intolerance, Dr. Peter Rowe has published a comprehensive science-based summary of best treatment (https://www.dysautonomiainternational.org/pdf/RoweOIsummary.pdf)

Preparing for Session 4

Before reading Session 4 on coping with stress and chronic illness, it is strongly recommended that you spend 2 weeks noting the events in your life that you find stressful and how those stressors impact your health. Remember that stress is very individual. Something that you might handle easily (or may have before you became ill) may be challenging to others or to the "new you." The information you record is for your own use, so try to be as detailed and honest as possible. You can only solve problems after you have identified them.

You will need the following:

- Adapted Karnofsky Energy Rating Scale
- Sleep Chart

To chart your daily stress levels, you will be using the pain column on the Sleep Chart to record stress on a scale of 1 (lowest) to 10 (highest), instead of pain.

Joan's Sleep Chart

Prior to this charting period, Joan made two changes. She noticed that her sleep initiation time was very long and talked to her family physician about something to help with that. The doctor prescribed zopiclone, a short-acting drug that helps people fall asleep faster. Joan also noted in her charting that she was often aware of noise during the night. She bought some silicone earplugs and uses them each night.

These two changes seem to have helped Joan's sleep. She is now falling asleep faster and reported no disruptions due to noise. Her sleep was not necessarily deeper (zopiclone does not increase sleep depth), but she had slightly increased sleep in the first part of the night, and as a result, her morning refreshment improved from mostly poor to mostly fair.

Name Joan Smith **Date** Jan 2 /12 **to** Jan 15/12
Meds: amitriptyline 20 mg NEW zopiclone 7.5 mg + earplugs
Supps: multi min / multi vit

Date	% Energy	~~Pain~~ Stress	Activities/other factors	HS Meds	Initiate mins	Depth	Aware	wake #/min	deep/ light	Refresh -ment
J2	55	3	work 4 hrs	Ami 20p	20	4	T, P	1/30	5/3	F
3	65	7	father to emergency	↓	20	4	D, P	—	7	P
4	50	8	mtgs at hospital		60	3	D, P	2/60	3/4	P
5	45	6	work 4 hrs		30	4	T	1/30	5/3	F
6	50	6	visit father, rest		30	3	T, P	2/60	4/3	P
7	55	5	errands, hospital		20	3	T	1/30	4/4	F
8	60	5	church, dinner with mother		30	3	—	1/20	5/3	F
9	65	4	work 4 hrs		20	4	T	1/30	5/3	F
10	65	4	go to look at care facilities		20	4	P	2/50	4/3	F
11	60	3	REST!		15	4	—	1/20	5/4	F+
12	65	3	work 4 hrs		30	3	P, T	1/30	4/3	F
13	60	8	call from LTD		70	3	P/T	3/70	3/3	P
14	45	8	paperwork		60	3	P/T	2/60	4/3	P
15	50	7	church, hospital	↓	40	3	P	1/40	4/3	P

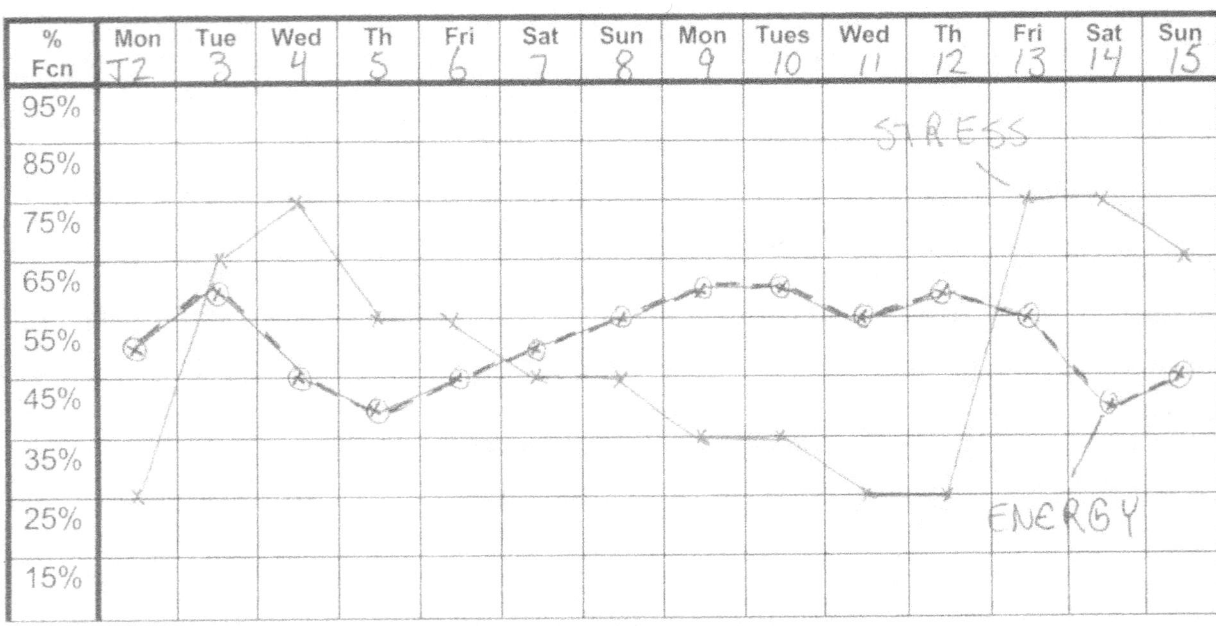

Adapted from the "sleep sheet" of Dr. Beverley Tompkins, Burke Institute, Calgary

Session 3 References

Appelman, B., Charlton, B.T., Goulding, R.P., Kerkhoff, T.J., Breedveld, E.A., Noort, W., . . . Wüst, R.C.I. (2024). Muscle abnormalities worsen after post-exertional malaise in long COVID. *Nature communications, 15*(1), 17. doi:https://www.nature.com/articles/s41467-023-44432-3

Bazelmans, E., Bleijenberg, G., van der Meer, J.W., & Folgering, H. (2001). Is physical deconditioning a perpetuating factor in chronic fatigue syndrome? A controlled study on maximal exercise performance and relations with fatigue, impairment and physical activity. *Psychological Medicine*, 31, 107-114.

Benrud-Larson, L.M., Dewar, M.S., Sandroni, P., Rummans, T.A., Haythornthwaite, J.A., & Low, P.A. (2002). Quality of life in patients with postural tachycardia syndrome. *Mayo Clin.Proc.*, 77, 531-537.

Brosseau, L., Wells, G.A., Tugwell, P., Egan, M., Wilson, K.G., Dubouloz, C.J., Casimiro, L., Robinson, V.A., McGowan, J., Busch, A., Poitras, S., Moldofsky, H., Harth, M, Finestone, H.M., Nielson, W., Haines-Wangda, A., Russell-Doreleyers, M., Lambert, K., Marshall, A.D., & Veilleux, L. (2008a). Ottawa Panel evidence-based clinical practice guidelines for aerobic fitness exercises in the management of fibromyalgia: part 1. *Phys.Ther.*, 88, 857-871.

Brosseau, L., Wells, G.A., Tugwell, P., Egan, M., Wilson, K.G., Dubouloz, C.J., Casimiro, L., Robinson, V.A., McGowan, J., Busch, A., Poitras, S., Moldofsky, H., Harth, M., Finestone, H.M., Nielson, W., Haines-Wangda, A., Russell-Doreleyers, M., Lambert, K., Marshall, A.D., & Veilleux, L. (2008b). Ottawa Panel evidence-based clinical practice guidelines for strengthening exercises in the management of fibromyalgia: part 2. *Phys.Ther.*, 88, 873-886.

Carruthers, B.M., Jain, A.K., De Meirleir, K., Peterson, D.L., Klimas, N., Lerner, A.M., . . . van de Sande, M.I. (2003). Myalgic Encephalomyelitis/Chronic Fatigue Syndrome: Clinical working case definition diagnostic and treatment protocols - A consensus document. *Journal of Chronic Fatigue Syndrome, 11*(1), 7–116.

Chu, L., Valencia, I.J., Garvert, D.W., & Montoya, J.G. (2018). Deconstructing post-exertional malaise in myalgic encephalomyelitis/ chronic fatigue syndrome: A patient-centered, cross-sectional survey. *PLoS ONE [Electronic Resource], 13*(6), e0197811. doi:https://dx.doi.org/10.1371/journal.pone.0197811

Eckey, M., Li, P., Morrison, B., Bergquist, J., Davis, R.W., & Xiao, W. (2025). Patient-reported treatment outcomes in ME/CFS and long COVID. *Proceedings of the National Academy of Sciences of the United States of America, 122*(28), e2426874122. doi:https://dx.doi.org/10.1073/pnas.2426874122

Edmonds, M., McGuire, H., & Price, J. (2004). Exercise therapy for chronic fatigue syndrome. *Cochrane. Database.Syst.Rev.*, CD003200.

Furlan, R., Jacob, G., Snell, M., Robertson, D., Porta, A., Harris, P., & Mosqueda-Garcia, R. (1998). Chronic orthostatic intolerance: a disorder with discordant cardiac and vascular sympathetic control. *Circulation*, 98, 2154-2159.

Germain, A., Giloteaux, L., Moore, G.E., Levine, S.M., Chia, J.K., Keller, B.A., . . . Hanson, M.R. (2022). Plasma metabolomics reveals disrupted response and recovery following maximal exercise in Myalgic Encephalomyelitis/Chronic Fatigue Syndrome. *JCI insight*. doi:https://insight.jci.org/articles/view/157621

Goudsmit, E. & Howes, S. Pacing: An alternative strategy to manage fatigue in CFS. 2007.

Goudsmit, E.M., Nijs, J., Jason, L.A., & Wallman, K.E. (2011). Pacing as a strategy to improve energy management in myalgic encephalomyelitis/chronic fatigue syndrome: a consensus document. *Disabil.Rehabil.*, 19**.**

Harvey, S.B., Wadsworth, M., Wessely, S., & Hotopf, M. (2008). Etiology of chronic fatigue syndrome: testing popular hypotheses using a national birth cohort study. *Psychosom.Med.*, 70, 488-495.

Hoel, F., Hoel, A., Pettersen, I.K., Rekeland, I. G., Risa, K., Alme, K., . . . Tronstad, K.J. (2021). A map of metabolic phenotypes in patients with myalgic encephalomyelitis/chronic fatigue syndrome. *JCI insight, 6*(16), 23. doi:https://dx.doi.org/10.1172/jci.insight.149217

Ichise, M., Salit, I.E., Abbey, S.E., Chung, D.G., Gray, B., Kirsh, J.C., & Freedman, M. (1992). Assessment of regional cerebral perfusion by 99Tcm-HMPAO SPECT in chronic fatigue syndrome. *Nuclear Medicine Communications*, 13, 767-772.

Jason, L., Benton, M., Torres-Harding, S., & Muldowney, K. (2009). The impact of energy modulation on physical functioning and fatigue severity among patients with ME/CFS. *Patient.Educ.Couns.*

Jason, L.A., Torres-Harding, S., Friedberg, F., Corradi, K., Njoku, M.G., Donalek, J., Reynolds, N., Brown, M., Weitner, B.B., Redemaker, A., & Papernik, M. (2007). Non-pharmacologic interventions for CFS: A randomized trial. *Journal of Clinical Psychology in Medical Settings*, 14, Dec-296.

Jones, K.D. & Clark, S.R. (2002). Individualizing the exercise prescription for persons with fibromyalgia. *Rheum.Dis.Clin.North Am.*, 28, 419-4xi.

Kindlon, T. (2011). Reporting of Harms Associated with Graded Exercise Therapy and Cognitive Behavioral Therapy in Myalgic Encephalomyelitis/Chronic Fatigue Syndrome. *Bulletin of the IACFS/ME*, 19, 59-111.

Lane, R.J., Barrett, M.C., Taylor, D.J., Kemp, G.J., & Lodi, R. (1998). Heterogeneity in chronic fatigue syndrome: evidence from magnetic resonance spectroscopy of muscle. *Neuromuscular Disorders*, 8, 204-209.

Larson, B.D., T.E.; Stevens, S.R.; Stevens, J.; Van Ness, J.M.; Snell, C.R. (2018). Reproducibility of Measurements Obtained During Cardiopulmonary Exercise Testing in Individuals With Fatiguing Health Conditions: A Case Series. *Cardiopulmonary Physiotherapy Journal*, 1–8.

Light, A.R., White, A.T., Hughen, R.W., & Light, K.C. (2009). Moderate Exercise Increases Expression for Sensory, Adrenergic, and Immune Genes in Chronic Fatigue Syndrome Patients But Not in Normal Subjects. *J.Pain*.

Light, K.C., White, A.T., Tadler, S., Iacob, E., & Light, A.R. (2012). Genetics and Gene Expression Involving Stress and Distress Pathways in Fibromyalgia with and without Comorbid Chronic Fatigue Syndrome. *Pain Res.Treat.*, 2012:427869. Epub; 2011 Sep 29., 427869.

Lund, E., Kendall, S.A., Janerot-Sjoberg, B., & Bengtsson, A. (2003). Muscle metabolism in fibromyalgia studied by P-31 magnetic resonance spectroscopy during aerobic and anaerobic exercise. *Scand.J.Rheumatol.*, 32, 138-145.

Marks, D.F. (2017). Special issue on the PACE Trial. In: SAGE Publications Sage UK: London, England.

Matthees, A., Kindlon, T., Maryhew, C., Stark, P., Levin, B. (2016). *A preliminary analysis of 'recovery' from chronic fatigue syndrome in the PACE trial using individual participant data.* Retrieved from https://www.virology.ws/wp-content/uploads/2016/09/preliminary-analysis.pdf

National Institute for Health and Care Excellence. (2021). *Myalgic Encephalomyelitis (or Encephalopathy)/ Chronic fatigue syndrome: diagnosis and management. NICE guideline [NG206*. Retrieved from https://www.nice.org.uk/guidance/ng206

Newton, J.L., Okonkwo, O., Sutcliffe, K., Seth, A., Shin, J., & Jones, D.E. (2007). Symptoms of autonomic dysfunction in chronic fatigue syndrome. *Quarterly Journal of Medicine*, 100, 519-526.

Newton, J.L., Sheth, A., Shin, J., Pairman, J., Wilton, K., Burt, J.A., & Jones, D.E. (2009). Lower Ambulatory Blood Pressure in Chronic Fatigue Syndrome. *Psychosom.Med.*

Nijs, J., Paul, L., & Wallman, K. (2008). Chronic fatigue syndrome: an approach combining self-management with graded exercise to avoid exacerbations. *J Rehabil.Med*, 40, 241-247.

Smith, M.B., Nelson, H.D., Haney, E., Pappas, M., Daeges, M., Wasson, N., & McDonagh, M. (2016). *Diagnosis and treatment of myalgic encephalomyelitis/chronic fatigue syndrome.*

Stevens, S., Snell, C., Stevens, J., Keller, B., & VanNess, J.M. (2018). Cardiopulmonary Exercise Test Methodology for Assessing Exertion Intolerance in Myalgic Encephalomyelitis/Chronic Fatigue Syndrome. *Frontiers in Pediatrics, 6*, 242. doi:https://dx.doi.org/10.3389/fped.2018.00242

Stewart, J.M. & Weldon, A. (2000). Vascular perturbations in the chronic orthostatic intolerance of the postural orthostatic tachycardia syndrome. *J Appl.Physiol*, 89, 1505-1512.

Stordeur, S., Thiry, N., & Eyssen, M. (2008). Syndrome de Fatigue Dhronique: diagnostic, tratiement et organisation des soins. (English Summary). 1-148. Bruxelles, Centre federal d'expertise des soins de sante (KCE). KCE Reports.

Streeten, D.H. & Bell, D.S. (1998). Circulating blood volume in chronic fatigue syndrome. *Journal of Chronic Fatigue Syndrome*, 4.

van Campen, C.L., Verheugt, F.W.A., Rowe, P.C., & Visser, F.C. (2020). Cerebral blood flow is reduced in ME/CFS during head-up tilt testing even in the absence of hypotension or tachycardia: A quantitative, controlled study using Doppler echography. *Clinical Neurophysiology Practice, 5*, 50–58. doi:https://dx.doi.org/10.1016/j.cnp.2020.01.003

Vernon, S.D., Funk, S., Bateman, L., Stoddard, G.J., Hammer, S., Sullivan, K., . . . Komaroff, A.L. (2022). Orthostatic Challenge Causes Distinctive Symptomatic, Hemodynamic and Cognitive Responses in Long COVID and Myalgic Encephalomyelitis/Chronic Fatigue Syndrome. *Frontiers in Medicine, 9*, 917019. doi:https://dx.doi.org/10.3389/fmed.2022.917019

White, P.D., Goldsmith, K.A., Johnson, A.L., Potts, L., Walwyn, R., DeCesare, J.C., Baber, H.L., Burgess, M., Clark, L.V., Cox, D.L., Bavinton, J., Angus, B.J., Murphy, G., Murphy, M., O'Dowd, H., Wilks, D., McCrone, P., Chalder, T., & Sharpe, M. (2011). Comparison of adaptive pacing therapy, cognitive behavior therapy, graded exercise therapy, and specialist medical care for chronic fatigue syndrome (PACE): a randomised trial. *Lancet.*, 377, 823-836.

Wilshire, C.K., T.; Alem Matthees & Simon McGrath (2016). Can patients with chronic fatigue syndrome really recover after graded exercise or cognitive behavioral therapy? A critical commentary and preliminary re-analysis of the PACE trial,. *Fatigue: Biomedicine, Health & Behavior, 5*(1), 43–56. doi: https://www.tandfonline.com/doi/full/10.1080/21641846.2017.1259724#d1e239

Wirth, K., & Scheibenbogen, C. (2020). A Unifying Hypothesis of the Pathophysiology of Myalgic Encephalomyelitis/Chronic Fatigue Syndrome (ME/CFS): Recognitions from the finding of autoantibodies against ß2-adrenergic receptors. *Autoimmunity Reviews, 19*(6), 102527. doi:https://doi.org/10.1016/j.autrev.2020.102527

Yamano, E., Watanabe, Y., & Kataoka, Y. (2021). Insights into Metabolite Diagnostic Biomarkers for Myalgic Encephalomyelitis/Chronic Fatigue Syndrome. *International Journal of Molecular Sciences, 22*(7), 26. doi:https://dx.doi.org/10.3390/ijms22073423

Session 4

Coping with Chronic Illness

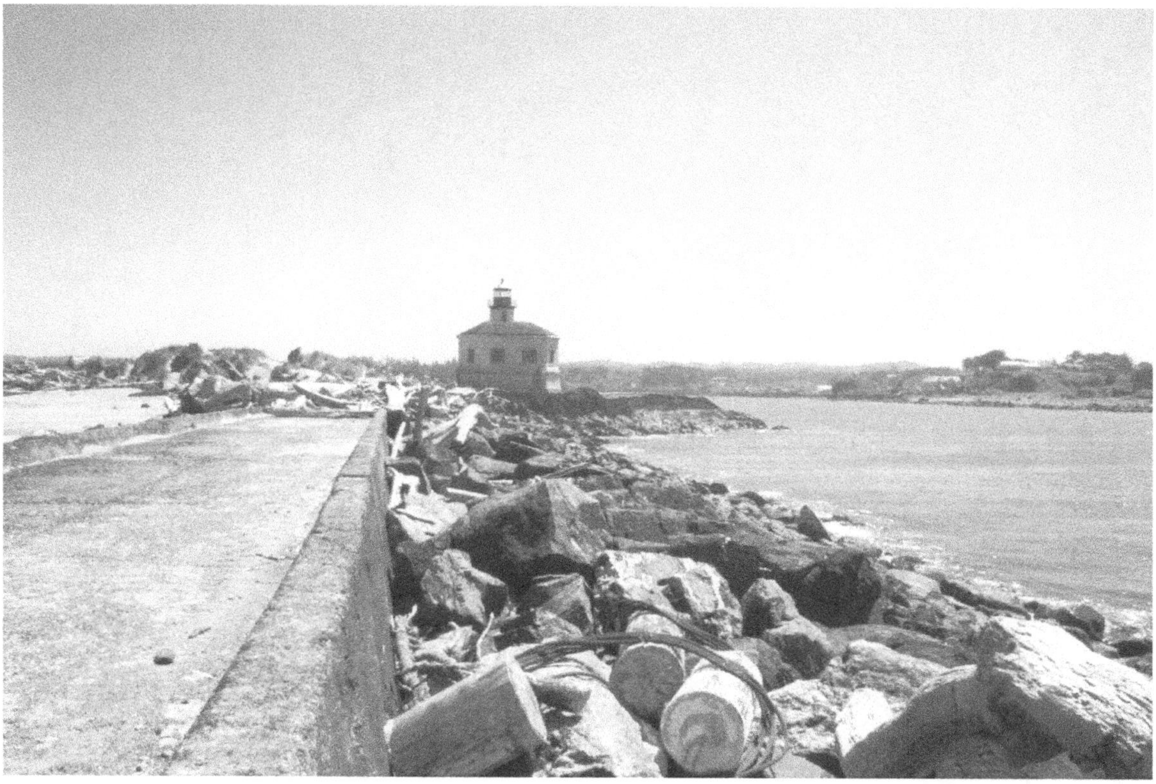

Travelling Down the Road to Wellness

We are all on a road to wellness and we are travelling down it.
There are a lot of us making the journey, the journey is not easy.
The symptoms are still there, sharply defined now.
We are taking action. It's very hard work.
We can see a path, we can see the target.
It's distant, dark and hazy, but we can see it.
We are learning how to manage our symptoms.
It seems overwhelming but we are working at it.
Will we ever get there?

The Road Well Travelled Part II

Session 4

Coping With Chronic Illness

Objectives

- To understand how the mind and the body are connected.
- To increase knowledge about coping with chronic illness.
- To improve stress management skills.
- To increase psychological empowerment.

The Biopsychosocial Model of Disease

We are much more than our bodies. We also have minds, feelings, families, relationships, and more. The physical severity of a medical condition is insufficient to predict an individual's illness experience. For example, the severity of changes visible on an X-ray or MRI is not a good predictor of the pain experienced by people with arthritis (Bedson & Croft, 2008). The biomedical (physical) model, invaluable in acute conditions, is not sufficient to explain the impact of chronic disorders.

In health and illness, there is a web of interaction between biology (the body), psychology (the mind) and the social environment (e.g., family function, social support, financial means, etc.). Hence, there is a need for another model that encompasses all factors that impact our health. All disease processes are influenced by psychosocial factors, including behavior, beliefs, experiences, relationships, and, for some, spiritual practice. This is true in chronic medical conditions such as cancer, arthritis, heart disease, and it is true in ME/CFS, FM and MCS.

In the field of complex chronic diseases, the term *biopsychosocial* has been misinterpreted and misused to invalidate people's lived experience. Biopsychosocial has become shorthand for “all in the head.” Biopsychosocial is not a zero-sum game. It reminds us that, in addition to the very real biomedical processes going on in chronic disease, there are other factors. It is not either/or. Recognizing all aspects of our complex lives in the formulation of why we feel as we do in any moment does not in any way invalidate the reality of the seriousness of the measurable biomedical abnormalities found in complex chronic diseases. The term biopsychosocial is a reminder that we are more than our bodies, not that our bodies are not important.

The biopsychosocial model of illness is complex and interactive and is significantly impacted by behavior. Health behavior has been defined as "an action taken by a person to maintain, attain, or regain good health and to prevent illness." Eating a healthy diet or stopping smoking are two examples of health behaviors.

A great deal of study has gone into understanding the factors that influence this behavior. We know that optimal adjustment to illness and disability is characterized by a broad range of factors, including subjective well-being, participation in meaningful activities, having satisfying relationships, and maintaining purpose and hope. This depends upon much more than measurable disability (e.g., immobility or pain). Health is an interaction between all aspects of a person. The suggestions in this manual are designed to help you optimize your health-related behaviors and attitudes, and through them, your health and well-being.

Personal Responsibility

Chronic disorders differ from acute conditions in that the patient bears much more responsibility for managing her/his/their condition. No doctor can fix or cure ME/CFS, FM or MCS with a pill. Although patients are not generally responsible for causing their condition, they are responsible for managing the condition. People with the ability to let go of the small stuff and who have effective problem-solving skills report greater acceptance of disability. Searching for and finding coping strategies, personal strengths, and family and social support assists adaptation. This is **your** job. No one else can do it for you, and you are capable of taking on this responsibility.

Impact of Life Events on ME/CFS and FM

Few studies have focused on the impact of stress and life events on people with ME/CFS and FM. I am not aware of any studies focused on the impact of live events in MCS. A recent study involving women with fibromyalgia, rheumatoid arthritis, or osteoarthritis showed that small negative daily life events have a negative impact on energy, while positive events have a very small or no impact on energy; in fact, some people became more tired even after positive events (Parrish et al., 2008).

A few studies report a connection between a life history of childhood sexual abuse and risk of developing both ME/CFS and FM. A few studies show that adult women with ME/CFS and FM are more likely than healthy women to have a history of childhood sexual abuse. Childhood sexual abuse is very stressful, and patients with many health conditions have this in their history.

I do not believe that there is a specific connection between ME/CFS, FM or MCS and childhood trauma. Childhood trauma is a huge stress on the body, and the impact of this stress is carried into adulthood. A history of childhood trauma predisposes all people to develop chronic health and mental health conditions. But this connection is no different in ME/CFS, FM or MCS than in other chronic conditions. The impact of childhood stress may eventually manifest in whichever body system an individual is most sensitive, due to genetic and other risks.

In some cases, the heart or the immune system may be affected. In the case of people with ME/CFS, FM or MCS, genetic predisposition to connective tissue laxity or altered immune function may be the weak link. In Session 8, I say a bit more about the connection between childhood abuse, anxiety disorders and ME/CFS and FM.

People with a history of childhood trauma or abuse may benefit from psychotherapy to help them come to terms with what has happened. If this describes you, please read the section below on "Psychotherapy: Is It for You?" And even if you do not have a history of childhood trauma, psychotherapy may, for other reasons, be a worthwhile option to consider.

Psychotherapy: Is It for You?

Being a psychiatrist with interest and training in psychotherapy, and having completed many, many years of psychotherapy myself, I have experienced the profound usefulness of therapy. At its best, psychotherapy offers a safe space in which to talk out loud about your history and/or your current situation. Doing this, especially when your story is witnessed and reflected by a compassionate professional who has no vested interest in your outcome, can be invaluable. You can gain perspective, compassion for yourself, confidence in your intuition, and develop ideas for change. It is said that much of the change that occurs in psychotherapy is not conscious. In other words, you don't have to know everything that's going on to benefit from it.

Safety First

But as I have said before, "any intervention with the power to help also has the power to hurt." Psychotherapy, if not conducted in a respectful, compassionate manner, can be extremely harmful. Therapists wield a lot of power and don't always use it for the benefit of their patients. If you sense that a therapist is too rigid in his or her beliefs or is not able to really hear your story, consider looking elsewhere.

Safety is paramount. All therapists should maintain clear boundaries between their professional and personal lives. You should not have the feeling that the therapist is using you to meet some need of his/

her/their own, other than the need to feel useful and to earn a living. It doesn't matter if a therapist is touted by others as being an expert. Your comfort and safety are more important.

If you have been seeing a therapist for several sessions and have no sense that you are progressing, you should bring it up for discussion. Maybe there is a reason intrinsic to your situation that will explain this, and maybe it will take time, but it is also possible that the approach isn't the right one for you. It takes a lot of courage to make the decision to leave a therapist and look for someone else.

Research shows that regardless of the therapeutic approach, the quality of the relationship between therapist and patient is the most important factor for change.

The Scope of Psychotherapy

What types of problems can therapy help with? Really, any thoughts, feelings, or behaviors that you believe hold you back from happiness and fulfillment can be addressed. These issues can extend from childhood or may have developed more recently. Many very emotionally healthy people continue to go for therapy at various times in life when they are facing a new challenge or an old one re-emerges. No problem is too large or too small. What is required is the emotional and physical time to devote to change, as well as the resources to pay for therapy.

Finding a Qualified Therapist

Some people are lucky enough to find a good therapist covered by insurance, but many are not. If you live in a location with GP psychotherapists, this may be an option. GP psychotherapists are general practitioners or family physicians who have devoted their practice to psychotherapy. Most have devoted many years to their own course of study in psychotherapy.

There are also some excellent therapists who work for the public health system and non-profit organizations. Sometimes they are limited in the amount of time they can spend with any one individual. But call around and see what your options are.

Another approach is to ask friends, family, or other professionals for referrals. Interview as many therapists as necessary until you find one who you feel will be a good fit for you. There are many paths to misery and many paths out.

The book *Living Well with a Hidden Disability: Transcending Doubt and Shame and Reclaiming Your Life* by Stacey Taylor and Robert Epstein has an excellent chapter on how to find a good therapist (Taylor, 1999). The book is out of print but still available through used book sellers. It is probably the most affirming book I have read on coping with conditions that cannot be seen or validated with tests. The bottom line is to trust your intuition.

Limitations of Psychotherapy

Psychotherapy isn't for everyone. Some people aren't interested in talking and don't benefit from it. Many studies have shown that people who benefit most from therapy are those who have relatively strong verbal skills and who are self-reflective. People who have at least one healthy, long-lasting relationship tend to do better than those who are extremely isolated. This probably reflects the centrality of the therapeutic relationship to the benefits of therapy. As well, the patient must be motivated to learn and change. Without this, regardless of how severe the problem or how skilled the therapist, success will be limited.

If you are considering therapy, remember that you should engage in therapy at the time that is right for you and not sign up just because you read here or elsewhere that it could be helpful. Similarly, the types of therapy that will work for you will be unique to your personality and experience. There are many effective approaches, ranging from ones that are very cognitive (focusing on thoughts) to approaches that focus on emotions and bodily sensations. Most useful therapies encourage increased self-awareness and learning or strengthening skills to deal with new and difficult situations.

Will Psychotherapy Improve My Physical Health?

People often wonder whether their physical health will improve if they go for psychotherapy. My response is that it is always better to resolve psychological issues than to leave them festering. All other things being equal, a person living in equanimity will have a better chance of improved health than one living in stress, anger, and resentment. But there is no guarantee that physical health will improve with therapy—ME/CFS, FM and MCS are complex and often mediated by factors that are difficult to change.

On the other hand, I am skeptical of psychological remedies for ME/CFS, FM and MCS that state or imply that "good thinking" can actually cure serious medical conditions. While a lucky few may improve, the majority will still be very ill despite developing a realistic, grateful, and hopeful attitude.

It is implied, but often not directly stated with these therapies, that people who are ill have somehow caused their conditions by their "wrong thinking." While unresolved stress and poor lifestyle choices can certainly impact health, I see many patients who do not seem to have contributed to their condition in any way. Patients have a big enough challenge to get better due to the complexity and severity of the illness. It is an unjust burden for them to have to also contend with other people's beliefs (or their own) that their illness is their fault.

Joan's Sleep/Stress Chart

For the discussion that follows, you'll need Joan's Sleep/Stress Chart and your own. During this charting period, instead of charting pain levels, Joan kept track of her stress levels. Two upsetting events happened. First, her father, who had been ill since before Christmas, had a setback and was admitted to the hospital. This meant that Joan had to add hospital visits and meetings regarding his care to her usual activities.

You can see that this stressor was associated with decreased energy. Joan recovered from this and began helping her mother with the process of looking at long-term care facilities and filling out the paperwork. Then Joan got a call from her long-term disability insurer, reminding her she needed to submit paperwork for her annual reassessment. Although Joan has been on LTD for a few years and is past the 2-year hurdle when many people lose coverage, any interaction with her insurer causes her to worry. After this phone call, her sleep was affected, and her energy dropped.

As you go through this chapter, look at Joan's Chart and look at your own. Can you identify any stressors from your charting? Try to identify both the stressors in your life and the impact they are having on your health. Remember that stress happens in life. But, for the most part, the impact that these inevitable events have is only negative if we let them be negative. The remainder of the session is devoted to information and tips on coping and stress management.

Coping

The Fennell Phase Model

Coping is a conscious effort to manage a stressful situation. Coping is not a constant. It changes over time and with experience. In the Coping Groups, which I facilitated for people struggling in this regard, we used Patricia Fennell's *The Chronic Illness Workbook* (Fennell, 2012). Check Fennell's website at http://www.albanyhealthmanagement.com/ on how to buy her book.

Fennell has created the *Four Phase Model* as a framework to help clinicians and patients comprehend and manage the process of coping with chronic illnesses. Similar to the well-known Kübler-Ross's stages of grieving, Fennell has described four phases of coming to terms with and managing chronic illness. **The phases are Crisis, Stabilization, Resolution, and Integration.**

Fennell's model allows for therapeutic intervention in a flexible phase-specific manner so that individuals may integrate their illness into a meaningful life despite physical limitations. The model is multimodal, addressing physical/behavioral, psychological, and social/interactive adaptation. The model recognizes that a patient's needs early in chronic illness may differ from the needs in later years, and may affect various responses to treatment, be it medical or psychosocial.

Fennell's model has been found to accurately describe the phases of illness adaptation that persons with ME/CFS go through (Jason et al., 2000). FM and MCS have not been similarly studied, but in my groups, the phase model seems to apply equally well to this population.

Fennell stresses that the four phases are not followed in a linear fashion; people move between phases, and aspects of more than one phase may be evident at any given time. Given the fluctuating nature of ME/CFS, FM, and MCS, there are always new challenges, and maintaining a *phase 4* or *integration* position is not a realistic goal. An alternative goal is to be flexible enough to adapt to the significant changes imposed by chronic illness.

Developing New Coping Strategies

One of the early lessons for people with ME/CFS, FM and MCS is that normal strategies of coping (i.e., working and trying harder and doing more) tend not to work. Many people, now ill, have successfully used these strategies earlier in their lives. This begs the question: Why doesn't it work this time?

The common answers are that people with ME/CFS, FM and MCS have fewer resources than they had before: less energy, less money, and often fewer friends and social supports. As well, the illnesses of ME/CFS and FM seem to change the ability to cope, possibly because of changes to the endocrine and autonomic nervous systems. Answers to the question as to why their former coping strategies do not work will be different for each person, and sometimes the answers are not forthcoming. The challenge is to learn new ways of coping and to accept that strategies that may have been successful in the past may not work with these illnesses.

The following questions are designed to help you re-evaluate your current coping strategies and see if you can find new ones to try. Writing the answers to these questions is often more helpful than just thinking about them. Please take the time to write your answers to at least the questions that seem important to you. Writing will force you to take the time to think through the answers and will allow you to go back to them later. You might be surprised by what you already know.

- What coping strategies do you attempt when you feel overwhelmed? Are these ones that used to work for you? Are these new strategies? Are the strategies working for you? If so, in what situations? Are there some situations in which they don't work? Can you think of different ways of managing those situations?
- What resources have you had in the past to rely on when you needed help? Can you still call upon these resources when needed? If not, can you think of some new ways to get these needs met?

- Since you became ill, have you had periods of stability (i.e., periods when you felt you were coping well)? If so, what did you do to contribute to that stability? Has something happened to change that now? What? What are some ideas you have that may help you get back to a more stable situation? Remember, you might not be able to change external events, but you can always change your reaction to events, no matter how upsetting or exciting.
- Do you ever blame yourself for your illness? If so, write out a list of what you did to contribute to your illness. Then list ways in which you have tried to lessen your condition. Which list carried more weight?
- If there are ways in which you contributed to some aspect of your condition (e.g., your health, your emotions, your social network, your family relations), how can you change your behaviors or attitudes so that these problems don't get worse? Remember, you can only change yourself, not anyone else. Putting energy into trying to change others may not be a good use of resources.
- Do you feel compassion towards yourself and your suffering? If not, what gets in the way?
- Are there any attitudes that you have learned from your family of origin, culture, or society that you will need to change to be respectful and compassionate toward yourself? It is possible that these attitudes were useful to you before, but are not now, given that your circumstances have changed. This often happens as people go through different life stages.
- Do you find yourself doing or saying things now that you never imagined you would do or say (for better or worse)? What are these things?
- What small actions do you take/could you take that would be an act of courage (i.e., standing for yourself)? Can you imagine how it would feel to stand up for yourself as much as you stand up for others?
- In what ways do you remain curious about life and what it has to offer? Are you acting on that curiosity? Even with your health limitations, could you take some steps in the direction of your curiosity?
- Can you imagine that you do not know all that life has to offer, that there may be something unexpected? Is there anything you can do to remain open to the unknown, to notice it, if it comes your way?
- Can you name one way in which you have changed or will change your priorities in life because of your illness?
- Can you name one thing you have learned from your illness that you may not have learned if you had remained healthy?
- Is there any way in which the illness experience has benefited you?

Grief

Grief is a universal issue for people with ME/CFS, FM and MCS. The losses/changes associated with these conditions are numerous and far-reaching. Likely, your life has changed significantly since becoming ill. Common losses include the following:

- Loss of financial and physical independence.
- Loss of your image of yourself as being a certain type of person.
- Changes in the role you play in your family and social network.
- Loss of support from family and friends who do not understand the illness.
- Loss of confidence in your ability to think.
- Loss of self-esteem from all the above.

How does a person cope with these? The good news is that it is possible (and even probable) that you will come to terms with these losses. The bad news is that it is impossible to arrive at resolution or acceptance except by going through grief. Grief means feeling and acknowledging the losses you have suffered, both due to illness and other losses in your life, even as you face an uncertain future. Grief involves the courage to step off one side of the cliff before knowing if you will get to the other side; letting go of the known and stepping into the unknown.

Acceptance

Acceptance is admitting the reality of your situation. It does not mean giving up on the future. Impermanence is the only constant in life, and we never know what is around the corner. If you learn as much as possible about your condition, the chances of positive change are greater than if you try to hide from that reality. An attitude of acceptance allows you to listen to your body and be kind to it (i.e., resting if tired, avoiding junk food, moderating exercise). It also involves facing and trying to solve problems that exist. Acceptance does not require endless worry about problems that cannot be changed. Rather, acceptance allows you to let go of problems you cannot solve, freeing up time to enjoy the moment as much as possible.

Non-Acceptance

Many people worry that paying too much attention to symptoms will make them worse. They fear that if they really allow themselves to recognize their vulnerability, they will fall into depression and not be able to climb back out. While it is true that over-focusing on the negative sucks joy out of life, rational appraisal of life does not.

Non-acceptance leads to people making the same mistakes over and over, hoping for a different result. The most common example of this is when people who don't face the severity of their physical limitation and get caught in a physical "crash and burn" cycle of constantly trying to do more than is possible, and crash as a result.

It is very painful to fully recognize the severity of loss of past and future opportunity caused by ME/CFS, FM and MCS. These disorders are chronic and can be severe and disabling. If you are shy about facing your reality, ask yourself what the alternatives are. What is likely to happen if you steadfastly deny and ignore what is happening to you?

Questions to Ask Yourself to Learn More About Your Grief

Each person's path through grief (coping with loss over which you have no control) is different. I cannot suggest the solutions, only help you focus on the questions that are the most concerning to you. The answers to some of these questions may reflect some unsolved dilemmas you are experiencing. Spending time with your personal dilemmas has the potential to lead to resolution.

If you feel really stuck and miserable, it may be a good time to seek professional help. I recommend writing the answers to these and other self-reflective questions.

- What have you accepted about your illness, and what have you not accepted?
- List the possible ways in which acceptance will help you and the ways in which non-acceptance will help you. Which list is longer and more compelling?
- Make a list of the losses/changes you have noticed as a result of your illness.
- What is the most difficult loss/change for you about being ill? Can you change any of those losses? If not, could you change your thinking about them so that they are less painful?
- Are there any losses/changes you feel you can't live with or accept?
- Can you change the things that you can't accept?
- If you can't change the loss and you can't accept it, what are your options?
- Do you listen to the messages your body sends you? When you listen, what happens? When you do not listen to your body, what happens?
- Which approach seems to work better for you in the short term? In the long term?

Finding Meaning

A common problem with chronic illness is feeling that life feels meaningless or useless when you cannot DO as much as you used to. Equating value with DOING is a culturally based assumption in the West. Other cultures (e.g., Hindu and Buddhist) place a much higher value on obtaining equanimity, wisdom, and compassion; traits that require mindfulness and BEING rather than DOING.

Making a shift from a DOING to a BEING value system is challenging since in our society, BEING doesn't receive much positive reinforcement. To make the transition, it is helpful to have self-confidence. By this, I mean having the confidence to take a step, even if it is not supported by those around you. Maybe you have had confidence in the past, maybe not. Your illness may give you the push to develop it more fully.

It is difficult to believe in things that are not tangible; that you cannot see, touch, or hear. However, if you think about what has been most important in your life, it is usually the intangibles that come to mind. Examples of intangibles include: a kind word, loving touch, note or phone call during a hard time, or someone who made an effort to understand. These acts of kindness and compassion are possible for all of us, even for the most severely ill.

In searching for small hints of meaning, it seems to help a lot to focus on what you can do rather than on what has been taken away. By seeing a cup as half full rather than half empty, one isn't lying to oneself, only viewing life from a different perspective, the perspective of self-affirmation and value. Why not choose this perspective over the alternatives?

Just as it is recommended for people with depression to keep a gratitude journal, I recommend keeping a “meaning” journal. Each day, write down one meaningful thing that has happened to you or that you have done. It can be as small as the pleasure of a new snowfall or as large as being there for someone on the edge of not being. If you keep track of how you focus on BEING in your life, your meaning in life may become clearer to you.

For people who are used to feeling control over their lives, grieving and finding meaning are very difficult. You cannot impose a meaning on your life as easily as when you were healthy. You may have to actively look for glimpses of meaning, sometimes in unexpected places.

Empowerment

As with all chronic medical conditions, long-term health status for people with ME/CFS, FM and MCS depends upon their ability to observe and trust the body's reactions to psychological and physical stressors, experimenting to see what works best and then making changes accordingly.

Self-management, as we talked about in Session 1, is accepted as the most cost-effective and successful approach to managing chronic illness.

The model of self-management developed by Kate Lorig and colleagues at Stanford School of Medicine is used worldwide. One of these courses, *Better Choices Better Health,* is a 6-week peer-led self-management group based on the work of Kate Lorig and her colleagues at Stanford University (Lorig et al., 2007).

Whether one is reading this manual, getting support online, or reading a self-help book, changes in emotional well-being occur when you experience a moment of realization regarding the validity of your own opinions. When you realize that your intuition is accurate and to be trusted, you stop searching for answers outside yourself. Yes, this means you have the answers within you! Outside information, such as in this manual, can assist you by encouraging you to think things through and view yourself from a different perspective, but it cannot give you the answers that will work for you.

You need to find your own path of recovery. Somewhere along your path, you will realize that you are not to blame for your disorder. Even if it were true that you contributed to being ill by overwork and/or over-worry, be aware that others also have these tendencies and have not paid the price you have paid. You have equal value and rights as others, despite your illness. When people recognize these few truths, they cope better, even if their physical condition or life circumstances do not improve.

Stress Management

Stress is experienced when a person's inner and outer resources are insufficient to deal with a problem or (more often) a series of problems. Inner resources include beliefs, confidence, problem-solving skills, and social skills. External resources include social support, material resources, legislation, public assistance, and cultural attitudes.

How stress is viewed affects a person's ability to cope with it. If a stressor is appraised as threatening or harmful, a person will be easily overwhelmed. Conversely, if a stressor is viewed as a challenge or an opportunity for change, a person is more likely to find a way to cope with it.

In the Canadian Consensus Definitions for ME/CFS, one manifestation of illness is the loss of adaptability and worsening of symptoms with stress. Homeostatic failures occur among patients with ME/CFS and FM. This means that the body cannot right itself the way it used to. For people with these conditions, small physical stressors such as walking up a flight of stairs or being in a cold room can cause exhaustion, pain, and other symptoms that can last for hours or days. Psychological stressors, such as interpersonal issues, which were easily managed before becoming ill, can feel monumental.

In part, this reaction may be due to circumstances over which patients have little control, and which may not be easily resolved. But there also seem to be physiological changes that make recovery from even small stressors difficult. The changes to the autonomic nervous system (discussed in Session 3) may have a role in this. For healthy people, many problems in life can be solved by making more effort or spending more money. However, patients with ME/CFS, FM and MCS are often short on both resources. As a result, their reserve for coping with stress is decreased. Therefore, patients' need for basic stress-management skills is greater than that for healthy people who have more reserve capacity.

Managing the Body

Managing stress entails managing the body and the mind. There are many strategies to cope better with stress. Any approach that assists the body in being relaxed, even in the face of ongoing stress, will be useful. Meditation, visualization, and breathing techniques are all useful strategies. When these are studied, it turns out that they all strengthen the parasympathetic arm of the autonomic nervous system.

You will recall from Session 3 that the parasympathetic nervous system is also called the *relaxation response*. And we have seen in *Session 2: Sleep Management* that turning down the sympathetic system has a role there, too. When working optimally, the parasympathetic nervous system allows blood pressure and heart rate to be lower (relaxed) and heart rate variability is enhanced. This variability in heart rate and strength is necessary for the body to respond to small changes in need from moment to moment. Very few interventions increase parasympathetic tone. Exercise is one of the best, but many people with ME/CFS and FM are limited in their ability to exercise. Meditation, relaxation, and deep breathing are alternatives for those in this situation.

If you have a spiritual practice, you may be able to find useful training through your spiritual group. If not, you might want to seek a course on *Mindfulness-Based Stress Reduction* (MBSR). This is an approach developed by Dr. Jon Kabat-Zinn specifically for use in a health care setting. MBSR has been shown to improve health status in patients with several serious chronic conditions, including chronic pain and psychiatric conditions such as depression. Information about MBSR, including a list of references and how to access study materials, can be found at the University of Massachusetts Medical School website: https://www.ummhealth.org/services-treatments/center-mindfulness/mindfulness-programs/mbsr. MBSR is a non-religious approach to meditation taught worldwide.

For breathing exercises, there are many options. One easily accessible is promoted by Dr. Andrew Weil (https://www.drweil.com/health-wellness/body-mind-spirit/stress-anxiety/three-breathing-exercises-and-techniques/).

The yoga tradition incorporates meditation, breathing, and body movement. It has a lot to offer, though I am not familiar enough with it to make recommendations. Some of my patients benefit from restorative yoga, a very gentle form developed to help people with injuries or illnesses. However, some find even this very gentle approach too exhausting. As with everything else, you should follow your intuition and try this approach if it appeals to you. If you do so, ensure you find a teacher who understands the limitations of people with your condition. And if it makes you feel worse instead of better, have the courage to stop.

Managing the Mind

A core strategy for managing the worry and stress feelings that accompany your life situation is to use your limited energy for solving problems that are solvable and put aside worries about things that cannot be changed. This is easily said and hard to do, but certainly possible. Here are some suggestions that may help lessen the number of things you have to keep in mind:

- Believe in yourself; your intuition has gotten you this far.
- Note and address thought patterns that are counterproductive. Try to identify where those thoughts came from. Stand back to get a broader perspective. This approach will be discussed further in the next section on Cognitive Behavioral Therapy.
- Use self-talk to get through hard times. Talking out loud can be very effective and may even bring a smile to your face (this from a psychiatrist).
- Learn about your personal boundaries. For example, how often do you do things you really don't want to do and then resent them afterwards?
- Learn assertiveness skills so that you can clearly communicate to others what is important to you.
- Use written reminders for tasks and messages to avoid confusion and errors.
- Prioritize and then delete the task with the least priority from your list—maybe it isn't that important.
- If the above suggestion brings terror (what if I take this task off my list and it turns out to be critical to my survival?), maybe you need to spend more time evaluating your priorities. To lessen your stress, it can help to match the tasks you have to do with the amount of energy you have to do them.

Is It Life Threatening?

In a previous group session, we began playing with questions to ask oneself when feeling overwhelmed. In her book *Kids Are Worth It*, parenting expert Dr. Barbara Coloroso asks parents to consider whether the natural consequences of a child's behavior are life-threatening, morally threatening, or unhealthy.

If none of these are true, she advises allowing children to learn from the natural consequences of their behavior rather than nagging, reminding, and warning. Natural consequences are the best learning experiences for adults as well. Here are the questions the group came up with to ask oneself about a worry:

- Is it the truth?
- Is it urgent?
- Is it life-threatening?
- Is it personal?
- Can I laugh about this?
- Does it really matter?
- Will it matter in 5 years?

Answer the questions honestly and trust your instincts. I hope that you have as much fun answering these questions as we had making them up. Did I mention yet that laughter is so important? Being able to laugh at oneself and at life is a sign that you are on the coping path. Of course, you might be in the process of something that is, in fact, threatening, such as a heart attack. In this case, I would advise you to call 911 or the equivalent emergency service.

The Cognitive Behavioral Model

The premise of cognitive behavioral psychology is that there are strong interactions between thoughts, emotions, and behavior and that many of these interactions are unconscious. The theory further suggests that if you note and address negative or counterproductive thoughts and belief systems, behaviors, and emotions can and will change. Many of us are unaware of the impact of our habitual thoughts. Examples of habitual thoughts relevant to chronic illness include:

- "I brought this on myself; I deserve to suffer."
- "No one is interested in hanging out with someone as sick as I am."
- "I have nothing to offer others now that I am ill."
- "There is no hope of getting better."
- "Nothing about my life is worthwhile."

Do you recognize yourself in any of these? Take time to write a list of thoughts you have about your illness. You will need to make this list over several days to pick up some thoughts that are less frequent and those of which you are less aware. If you don't notice any negative thoughts, you can skip the rest of this section.

Note that not all patients have incorrect or counterproductive beliefs that are preventing recovery. Some patients amaze me with their determined optimism in the face of severe symptoms. Some beliefs are reality-based and not amenable to therapy. If your list of negative thoughts is very short, then cognitive approaches may not have much to offer you.

If you have identified negative thoughts, read on. Repetitively thinking thoughts that are blaming or disrespectful of yourself, even below the threshold of awareness, can impair your ability to get and feel better. To the extent that each of us has these types of thoughts, Cognitive Behavioral Therapy (CBT) can help.

There are excellent self-help books on CBT. I recommend any of the books by Dr. David Burns, including his best seller, *Feeling Good: The New Mood Therapy* (Burns, 2000). Burns' books are easy to read and have excellent exercises to help readers assess and change their thinking. Cognitive behavioral strategies are helpful for many things, including, but not limited to, becoming calmer, regulating mood, becoming more confident in social situations, and becoming less perfectionistic. The positive message of CBT is that change is possible even if your thoughts are ingrained over a lifetime.

The form of CBT described by Burns and others, and commonly used by therapists, is open-ended. This means that although the therapist will know the common negative thoughts that people with various conditions tell themselves, they do not assume what thoughts and behaviors a given individual will have. The process of CBT is collaborative. The therapist guides the patient in an examination of belief systems and behaviors.

A skilled therapist will guide the patient to envision alternative thoughts but is not directive. Many times, the therapist's assumptions are as incorrect as those of the patient. Psychotherapy is about becoming more open-minded and considering new ideas, not about taking on any particular belief system, especially that of your therapist, or beliefs that are overly optimistic or untrue.

This collaborative, non-directive form of CBT differs from the model developed for the treatment of ME/CFS by a group of British psychiatrists (the model that is used in several studies on CBT in ME/CFS) (Deale et al., 1997; Sharpe et al., 1996). The *British model* assumes that specific cognitive distortions feed maladaptive behavior that, in turn, perpetuates the specific symptoms of ME/CFS. This model suggests that patients with ME/CFS hold the inaccurate belief that their condition is physical in nature; cope ineffectively by avoiding activity; and have high symptom preoccupation. I'll say a bit more about this school of thought in Session 8. The CBT developed by Sharpe and others "aims to help the patient to recover by changing these unhelpful cognitions and behaviors" (Sharpe et al., 1996).

While I am always on the lookout for such mistaken beliefs, in 11 years of practice, I have rarely found these cognitions and behaviors to be "game changers." I find the opposite is more often true. Patients are more commonly not accepting of their limitations, and they push through severe symptoms, causing a relapse in health.

As a therapist, I find that having an *a priori* assumption about a person's attitudes and beliefs to be disrespectful and non-collaborative. I hope that when I make this error, my patients let me know.

Finding Balance: A Self-Reflection Exercise

Paediatrician Dr. Katherine Rowe is one of the most experienced ME/CFS doctors in the world. She has followed a cohort of child and adolescent patients in Melbourne, Australia, for over 20 years. The following exercise is inspired by her successful work with these young patients (Rowe & Rowe, K.J., 2000).

For this exercise, you will need paper and some coloured pencils. On the paper, draw two large circles, one on the top and one on the bottom of the sheet. Label the top circle *Actual Activity Percentages* and the bottom circle *Ideal Activity Percentages*. For a week or more, carefully observe yourself and note what percentage of waking hours you spend in the following activities:

- Necessary life tasks (things you **don't like** to do but have to do to survive, such as errands, cleaning, banking, phone calls with call centre computers, etc.).
- Work/school (you may or may not enjoy this).
- Necessary self-care (things that help you but take time and energy, such as charting, cooking healthy meals, and physical and mental stimulation).
- Appointments with professionals (do you really need to see so many professionals?).
- Family time.
- Social time.
- Fun/self-nurturing (e.g., reading a good book, sitting in nature, drawing, playing music, talking to a close friend).

Note that some of the categories may overlap (e.g., family time can be either nurturing or stressful; work can be stressful or affirming). Spend some time choosing categories that are most meaningful to you. Then choose a colour that represents your feelings about each category. For example, give your favourite category your favourite colour or a colour that represents that activity.

Now return to the page with the two circles. Roughly calculate from your diary the percentage of time each day that you spend in each activity type, including resting during the day. Record this as a pie chart, colouring in each segment with a different colour so that it is easy to notice how you spend your time.

If, for example, you spend 50% of your time in a certain activity, you will have 1/2 of your pie coloured in the colour representing that activity.

Now, on the bottom circle, create an "ideal" pie chart. Given that each of us has certain necessary tasks and responsibilities, and given your current health status, how would you like your life balance to look?

Now set a small, concrete, achievable goal to move your actual pie chart closer to your ideal. An example may be to schedule one fun thing (within your energy limitations) each week. Experiment with different ideas and note what activities help you feel best, physically, cognitively, and emotionally.

Remember that purposeful rests and naps are activities! Use this information to fine-tune your goals and make further changes so that you are able to enjoy your life more while still completing enough of the "have to activities." You may want to spend more time on this exercise before continuing with your preparation for the next session. Shaping your life to be closer to one that you will enjoy and gain meaning from is very important.

The diagram on the next page shows Joan's pie charts. You will see that in her life, she currently spends a lot of time going to appointments and doing household chores. Her goal is to increase the time available to spend with friends, family and for personal nurturing activities. She may be able to find this time if she goes to fewer appointments. This might be a long-term goal.

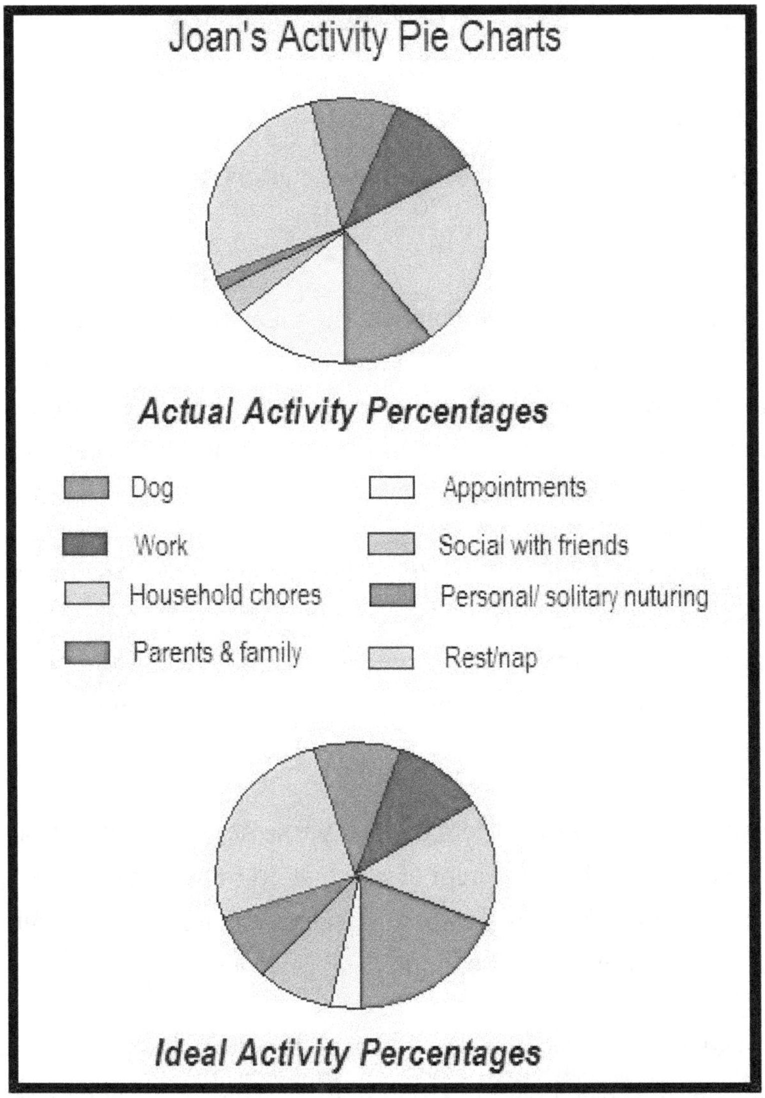

Preparing for Session 5

Before reading the next session on diet, it is strongly recommended that you complete a 10-Day Diet Diary. Diet changes from day to day. Therefore, it is important to record your intake for several days to get an accurate reflection of your typical nutritional intake and food choices. The Diet Diary is the most difficult and time-intensive homework in this manual. In my experience, those who complete the exercise find it, despite its difficulties, to be extremely important and worthwhile.

There are two ways to record your food intake: by pen and paper, or by using an online or purchased computer application.

If you choose to use pen and paper, you will require

- Daily Diet Diary: 10 copies.
- A book or online resource describing the nutritional content of food.
- A calculator.

First record each food you eat in the "Food" column. Then leave enough space so that you can record each ingredient of that food in the "Contents" column. Write the amount of each ingredient either by weight, if you have a scale, or by volume (e.g., 1 cup of oats). Then look up each ingredient in your information book or website and record how many grams of protein, fat, carbohydrate, and calories were contained in the serving size you consumed.

At the end of each day, tally the total for each column. It is also helpful to record the number of servings of fruits and vegetables each day, the amount of complete protein (protein from animal sources), and the volume that you drink. A serving size for fruit and vegetables is approximately 1/2 cup. At the end of 10 days, add the totals for each day together and divide by 10. This will give your average intake of each of the major nutrient categories.

If you choose to do your recording online, there are many free apps to choose from. For every food that you enter, apps typically give you a huge amount of information, including calories, protein, fat (including types of fat and cholesterol), carbohydrate content, as well as mineral, vitamin, amino acid and fatty acid content, glycemic load, and even inflammation index.

Choose the app that gives the information you are most interested in and is easy for you to use. To get the most out of the exercise, it is also helpful to record other symptoms, such as sleep, pain, etc., so that you can begin to notice connections between what you eat and your symptom profile.

Diet Diary Tips

When looking up a food you are eating in a calorie counter book or program, make sure that you note if it is cooked or raw.

- 1 cup of raw rice has 685 calories

- 1 cup of cooked rice has 169 calories
- 100 grams of raw chicken breast without skin has 110 calories
- 100 grams of roasted chicken breast without skin has 165 calories

Why the difference? 1 cup of raw rice cooks up into several cups of cooked rice. Raw meat has a lot of water content, almost 50% in some cases. The water decreases with cooking, leaving more nutrients per gram of meat.

Make sure to note the quantity of food that you are eating. On most packages, a serving size is defined and may not be the same as what you are eating.

For this exercise, precision is not critical. You don't need to weigh every ingredient to get an approximation of your intake. It is much better to get a ballpark idea of whether you need to make changes to your diet or not than to strive for perfection and not complete the exercise.

In my experience, virtually every group participant who takes the time to do this homework learns something useful about his/her/their diet. If you think you know enough about your diet, you are probably mistaken. The only people who may give this homework a pass are people with severe eating disorders, for whom this much focus on food eaten may throw them into a relapse. This is a small minority of people.

On the following pages are two of Joan's diet entries: first, a full day of intake, and second, a recipe that she made and ate over the next several days.

Daily Diet Diary

Date Feb 13/12 Name Joan Smith

Time	Food	Contents	Amount	Protein	Fat	Carbs	Cals
9:00	rye bread		1 slice	3g	1g	15g	82
	peanut butter		1 tbsp	8g	8g	6g	94
	honey		1 tbsp	∅	∅	17g	64
	coffee		1 cup	∅	∅	∅	2
3pm	pear		1 med.	1g	∅	13g	122
4pm	coffee		1 cup	∅	∅	∅	2
6pm	peas		1/2 cup	4g	∅	12g	66
	chicken	(no skin)	1/2 breast	27g	1g	∅	142
	scalloped potatoes	home made	1 cup	7g	9g	26g	216
8pm	microwave popcorn	1 bag	1 bag	2g	14g	15g	180
	banana		1 med	1g	∅	27g	105
				Protein	Fat	Carbs	Cals
Total				53g	33g	184g	1075

servings fruits 4 (1 serving = 1/2 cup) complete protein 27g

servings veg 1 litres water 1.5 l

Daily Diet Diary

Date Feb 15/12 Name Joan Smith

Time	Food	Contents	Amount	Protein	Fat	Carbs	Cals
	Split Pea Soup Recipe (entered in nutritiondata)						
	basil		2 tbsp	0	0	0	1
	carrots		4 med	4	0	24	100
	celery		4 stalks	0	0	8	40
	olive oil		2 T	0	28	0	238
	onion		1/2 raw	1	0	5	22
	split peas		1 lb	111	5	274	1547
	paprika		1 teasp.	0	0	1	6
	thyme		1 T	0	0	2	7
	chorizo (custom entry)		5 sausages	55	35	10	560
			total	173	67	322	2526
	If eaten in 6 servings	total / serving		29	11	54	421
				Protein	Fat	Carbs	Cals
Total				29	11	54	421

servings fruits Ø (1 serving = 1/2 cup) complete protein 9 g

servings veg ? are split peas a veg or a carb? litres water ~0.3

Session 4 References

Bedson, J., & Croft, P. R. (2008). The discordance between clinical and radiographic knee osteoarthritis: a systematic search and summary of the literature. *BMC Musculoskeletal Disorders, 9,* 116. doi:https://link.springer.com/article/10.1186/1471-2474-9-116

Burns, D. (2000). *Feeling Good: The New Mood Therapy,* pp. 1-706. Quill (Harper Collins), New York.

Deale, A., Chalder, T., Marks, I., & Wessely, S. (1997). Cognitive behavior therapy for chronic fatigue syndrome: a randomized controlled trial. *American Journal of Psychiatry*, 154, 408-414.

Fennell, P.A. (2012). *The Chronic Illness Workbook: Strategies and Solutions for Taking Back Your Life, revised edition.,* Albany Health Publishing, Albany, NY.

Jason, L.A., Fricano, G., Taylor, R.R., Halpert, J., Fennell, P.A., Klein, S., & Levine, S. (2000). Chronic fatigue syndrome: an examination of the phases. *J Clin Psychol.*, 56, 1497-1508.

Lorig, K., Halsted, H., Sobel, D., Laurent, D., Gonzalez, V., & Minor, M. (2007). *Living a Healthy Life with Chronic Conditions, Canadian Third Edition,* 3rd edn, Bull Publishing, Boulder, Colorado.

Parrish, B.P., Zautra, A.J., & Davis, M.C. (2008). The role of positive and negative interpersonal events on daily fatigue in women with fibromyalgia, rheumatoid arthritis, and osteoarthritis. *Health Psychol.*, 27, 694-702.

Rowe, K.S. & Rowe, K.J. (2000). Symptom Patterns in Children and Adolescents with Chronic Fatigue Syndrome. International Perspectives on Child and Adolescent Mental Health: Selected Proceedings of the Second International Conference on Child & Adolescent Mental Health, Kuala Lumpur, Malaysia, June 2000 (ed. by N. N. Singh, T. H. Ollendick, & A. N. Singh), pp. 395-422. Elsevier.

Sharpe, M., Hawton, K., Simkin, S., Surawy, C., Hackmann, A., Klimes, I., Peto, T., Warrell, D., & Seagroatt, V. (1996). Cognitive behavior therapy for the chronic fatigue syndrome: a randomized controlled trial. *BMJ*, 312, 22-26.

Taylor, S. (1999). *Living Well with a Hidden Disability: Transcending Doubts and Shame and Reclaiming Your Life,* pp. 1-272. New Harbinger, Oakland, California.

Session 5

Management of Diet and Gastrointestinal Symptoms

Out of the Fog

Towards Successful Management of ME/CFS, FM and MCS

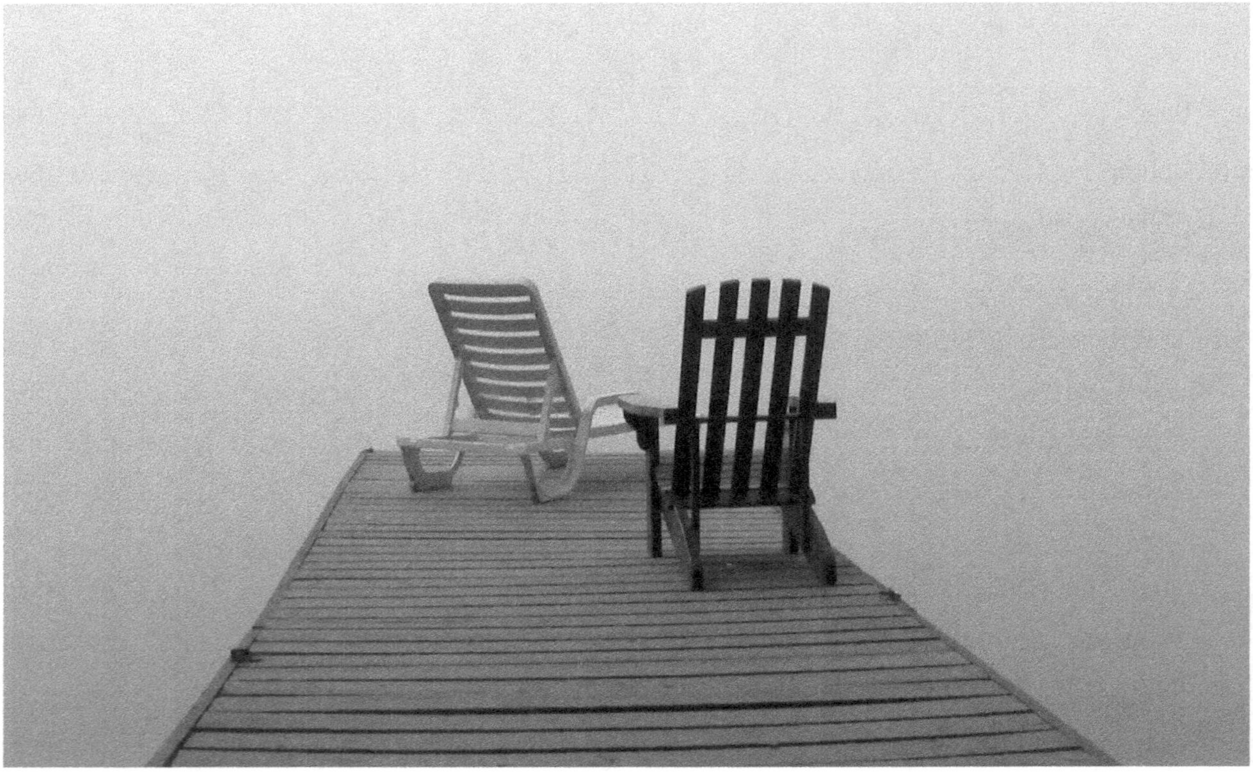

Angélique Wagner, Calgary, AB

Session 5

Management of Diet and Gastrointestinal Symptoms

Objectives

- To increase knowledge about nutrition needs in ME/CFS, FM and MCS.
- To learn to identify food-related health and mental health symptoms.
- To use diet to maximize nutrition and minimize symptoms.
- To identify and manage irritable bowel symptoms.

Introduction

There are two main topics in this session. The first is a discussion of nutritional issues for people with ME/CFS, FM and MCS. The second is the identification and management of gastrointestinal symptoms with a focus on irritable bowel syndrome (IBS), a condition commonly comorbid with ME/CFS, FM and MCS. Irritable bowel syndrome is included among the Canadian Consensus diagnostic criteria for both ME/CFS and is frequently comorbid with FM and orthostatic intolerance.

I am not a nutritionist or a gastroenterologist. Therefore, the information presented is not that of a specialist in the field but rather is based on what I have learned and observed in practice. Individual health status must be taken into account, and all recommendations should be discussed with your general physician, naturopathic doctor or dietitian before implementation.

Finding Dietary Advice

Diet is so controversial. There are strong opposing opinions, and finding a registered dietitian who understands complex chronic conditions can be difficult. Depending on your specific needs, be sure to ask about their knowledge of chronic illness, irritable bowel syndrome, and food allergies and sensitivities.

Before reading this section, I recommend gathering accurate information about your nutritional intake and identifying whether your symptoms are influenced by what you eat. A 10-Day Diet Diary (which you should have completed, following Session 4), recording all foods eaten with the calorie, protein, and fat content, gives an initial assessment of nutritional intake.

Joan's Diet Diary

One day of Joan's 10-Day Diet Diary and one of her recipes is included in Session 4 for illustration. To interpret her Diet Diary and calculate how much she needs to eat each day to maintain her health, Joan needs to calculate her recommended daily intake based on her size and activity level. How you can make these calculations for yourself will be explained in more detail later in this session under "adequate diet." Joan is 5 feet 4 inches tall. This means that her ideal weight is 120 lbs or 54 kg. Based on this weight and her relatively sedentary activity level, Joan's caloric intake should be about 1650 Kcalories per day. What we commonly call a *calorie* is actually a *kilocalorie, Kcalorie* or *Kcal*.

The tracking day shown in Session 4 was a workday for Joan. Apart from a pear during her break at work, Joan didn't eat between breakfast and supper. She may want to notice whether this affected any of her symptoms. Some people feel more tired if they don't eat for several hours in a row. Think about your own food intake and how it is spaced over the day.

In terms of total intake, Joan didn't eat much (1075 Kcalories) on that day, compared to her body's caloric needs of 1650 Kcalories. It may or may not have been a typical day for her. She will want to compare her energy and symptom levels on this day to other days in which she eats differently. As you read this chapter, notice how Joan did with regard to fruits and vegetables, the most nutritious food groups. Think about your own food intake in these food groups.

While keeping your Diet Diary, also record your daily health and mental health symptoms. This will tip you off to whether you are reacting adversely to any foods. People tend to look for gastrointestinal symptoms such as gas, bloating, indigestion, diarrhea, and constipation. However, foods can cause virtually any symptom, including pain, fatigue, depression, anxiety, and dizziness.

Don't assume which symptoms may be related to your diet. Keep an open mind and write everything down. Remember that many food-related symptoms are delayed, so you will need to record for days to weeks to notice patterns. If you think that food is affecting your symptoms, I recommend using the *Activity and Symptoms Chart*. Write what you eat in the activity column and your symptoms in the *symptoms* column. After several days of charting, you may begin to notice patterns.

Without carefully recorded information, you will be unable to judge what types of changes you should consider making to your diet. Each person is different, and following what has helped others may not work for you.

Part I. Dietary Issues in ME/CFS, FM and MCS

Several studies have suggested that people with ME/CFS, FM and MCS have nutritional deficiencies. However, the studies are small and not replicated. This means there is a large variation among individuals, and no "one size fits all" solution. You may or may not have dietary problems, and this can only be assessed by completing a 10 Day Diet Diary. Nutritional problems can only be accurately assessed through testing. Many of the useful tests listed in this session are not available through the Canadian public health care system. Refer to Session 1 for more information on how to access nutritional and other tests not offered or available through the Canadian public health care system.

Where they exist, nutritional problems may be related to the following:

1. Inadequate Diet.
2. Food choices.
3. Inadequate digestion.
4. Inadequate absorption.
5. Food sensitivities/allergies.
6. Dysbiosis (suboptimal bacterial ecology in the gastrointestinal tract).
7. Psychological factors.

Adequate Diet

Many patients who are chronically ill are too sick, tired, and poor to prepare fresh, healthy, diverse foods on a regular basis. For others, decreased appetite, nausea, and/or abdominal pain or irritable bowel syndrome lead to decreased food intake. Necessary intake depends on a whole range of factors, including size, gender, activity level, and health status. Most nutrition apps have tools to help you calculate your needed caloric intake while taking these important variables into account.

Ideal Weight

To calculate optimal nutritional intake, you must first determine your *ideal weight*. Ideal weight is the weight of healthy tissues (muscle, bones, organs, etc.) that need to be supported by the nutrition you consume. Note that *ideal body weight* is not the same, in most cases, as actual weight. Some people are under and some over this ideal weight. This weight is for the purpose of intake calculations. Your goal weight may differ from this number. Please don't get too depressed at this point if your ideal weight is far below what you think you can achieve.

An estimate of ideal weight can be calculated easily based on your height. If you are very fine-boned or big-boned, you will need to use a more sophisticated measurement. The general calculation is

- For women, start with 100 lbs for the first 5 feet of height. Add 5 lbs for every inch you are tall (above 5 feet). For example, a 5-foot-6-inch woman of medium build has an ideal weight of (100 + (5 x 6)) or 130 lbs.
- For men, start with 110 lbs for the first 5 feet of height. Add 6 lbs for every inch you are tall (above 5 feet). For example, a 5-foot-11-inch man of medium build has an ideal weight of (110 + (6 x 11)) or 176lbs.

Most calculations in nutrition use the metric system. To convert your weight in pounds (lbs) to kilograms (kg) for the following calculations, divide by 2.2 (e.g., an ideal weight of 130 pounds equals 59 kg). For ease of calculation, I recommend rounding up to 60 kg.

Daily Caloric Needs

For women: 30 Kcal/Kg Ideal Weight/day
For men: 35 Kcal/Kg Ideal Weight/day

- For a woman with an ideal weight of 60 kg, the recommended caloric intake will be 60 kg X 30 Kcal/Kg/day = 1800 Kcal/day. This is the intake required to maintain health if one's activity level is sedentary. Consult a website or book to calculate how to increase your needs calculation to reflect your activity level.
- A person with depleted nutritional stores or who is recovering from illness, injury, or surgery requires more food than someone who is healthy.
- Patients with ME/CFS, FM and MCS may require additional calories, especially those who are severely ill and/or those with significant indigestion or diarrhea. Surprisingly, some people begin to eat more and lose weight. This may be because increased intake allows the metabolism to increase.

Daily Protein Needs

1.5 g/Kg Ideal Weight/day

- Most nutrition guides emphasize that people in North America eat too much animal protein. The often-recommended amount is 1.0 g/Kg Ideal Weight/day. For a 60 kg woman, this equates to: 60 kg X 1.0 g/Kg/day = 60 g protein per day cooked weight.
- This amount **does not** include water, which comprises up to 50% of raw meat weight or fat.
- Some people with ME/CFS break down and excrete more muscle protein than healthy people (Dunstan et al., 2000). Therefore, the body may require more protein than is generally advised. I recommend 1.5 g/Kg Ideal Weight/day. For a 60 kg woman, this equates to: 60 kg X 1.5 g/Kg/day = 90 g protein per day cooked weight.
- Clinical experience with patients with ME/CFS, FM and MCS suggests that this protein should be split into at least three servings per day, and two of these servings should be from animal sources, such as meat, fish, eggs, or dairy. Animal protein is a complete protein, meaning that it has all of the amino acids that humans require to build new tissues.
- Though a vegetarian diet is recommended for some health conditions, such as heart disease and cancer, it does not work well for people with ME/CFS, FM and MCS. If you don't believe this, try decreasing your protein intake for several weeks and assess how you feel.
- Exceptions to this increased protein requirement are persons with gout, kidney disease, or disorders of protein metabolism or excretion. They should consult with their physician or dietitian before increasing protein intake.

Daily Fat Needs

1.0 g/Kg lean body mass/day

- For a 60 kg woman, 1g/Kg/day X 60 kg = 60 g fat per day.
- This is higher than is ideal for weight loss and decreased risk for heart disease and breast cancer. If you also need to consider these conditions, you may attempt a lower fat intake. Be aware, however, that you have to get your calories from some type of food. If you lower fat, you will likely increase carbohydrates, which increases the risk of metabolic syndrome (see below). Diet is a difficult balancing act, as you must account for all your health risks and needs. If your situation is complicated, consult a dietitian.
- Some fat will be eaten as part of animal protein (e.g., milk, eggs, meat, or fish). Any fat in addition to this should be "good" fat. "Good" fat refers to fat sources that don't significantly increase the risk of heart disease and stroke. This includes fat from raw nut and seed sources, including the essential fatty acids found in flax, fish, borage, and evening primrose oil.

The trans fats found in processed foods (hydrogenated oils) should be absolutely avoided. Trans fats are artificially altered to allow longer shelf time without spoiling. Any food on the inner aisles of the supermarket may have trans fats. Read all labels on prepared foods. Trans fats insert themselves into cell membranes, replacing normal, healthy fats. They don't act the same; they make the membranes stiffer, and as a result, receptors in the membrane don't work as well. All the nutrition in the world won't help if your cells can't communicate with each other and with their own nucleus and mitochondria.

It is becoming clear that the North American diet is high in omega-6 fatty acids and deficient in omega-3 fatty acids. Supplementation should include omega-3 fatty acids, but omega-6 and omega-9 fatty acids are rarely required. This means that the commonly purchased omega 3/6/9 mixes may not be the best nutritional choice. There are several types of omega-3 fatty acids. The two that most people are deficient in, eicosapentaenoic acid (EPA) and docosahexaenoic Acid (DHA), are present only in marine sources, such as fish oil. They can also be manufactured from marine algae.

Product: Omega-3 fatty acids from fish oil

Supplier: Nordic Naturals and others

Note: Omega-3 fatty acid supplements should be pharmaceutical grade and molecularly distilled to avoid contamination with mercury and polychlorinated biphenyls (PCBs), among other toxins. PCBs were once widely used in industry, are highly fat-soluble and concentrated in fish. Ingesting even tiny amounts of PCBs causes human health problems, including cancer. Quality testing of fish oil products is done at the University of Guelph, and test results are available online at https://certifications.nutrasource.ca/

Dose: The recommended daily dose of fish oil for nutrition and heart health is 2-4 capsules (500-750 mg/capsule).

Food Choices

Benefits of Real Food

There are thousands of naturally occurring substances in food that have a chemical and nutritional impact on the body for better or worse. For most of these substances, we have no nutritional information. Nutritional supplements provide only the molecules that we know are important, but not the hundreds that are yet to be identified. As a result, there is no substitute for unadulterated "real" food. Only a diet comprised of diverse, real foods gives adequate nutrition.

Some severely ill patients rely on commonly available meal replacement drinks. Most of these have an astounding amount of sugar in them and not enough of the critical nutrients. Read the labels for yourself if you don't believe me. No food replacement includes the hundreds of micronutrients that are found in real food. I strongly recommend not using these meal replacement products except for very occasional or emergency use (e.g., if you are not able to obtain or prepare any other food and are risking starvation).

Of course, finding, purchasing, and preparing real food is easier said than done, especially for the severely ill, for whom a trip to the grocery store takes all the allotted energy for a week. The optimal situation is to have someone to assist with shopping and preparing food. You might be able to ask a friend to pick up your list when he/she/they go shopping. Increasingly, grocery stores will deliver for a small fee.

Many people cook infrequently, making enough for several servings and then freezing portions for later use. I personally love my slow cooker. Put the ingredients in, go to bed, and voilà, a delicious meal is ready in the morning. If you sleep up to 12 hours a night, you have to be able to tolerate well-cooked food. Some people are able to find prepared frozen meals that meet their nutritional needs. If you go this route, be sure to read the label carefully to check for nutrition and unwanted additives.

Home care service providers are underfunded, and even the most severely ill patients are often unable to access in-home help with cooking and cleaning unless they can pay privately. It has been shown in the Canadian Community Health Survey that patients with ME/CFS, FM and MCS have more unmet health and home care needs and are more food insecure than most other Canadians with chronic disorders (Parlor, 2009). There is a need for improved funding of home care services and an increased awareness of the validity and severity of the needs of patients who are severely ill with ME/CFS, FM and MCS.

Benefits of Organic Food

The nutritional quality of food has changed dramatically in the past 60 years. Research shows that conventionally grown and produced food contains measurable amounts of hormones, antibiotics, herbicides, and pesticides, as well as preservatives and chemicals to enhance color, texture, etc. These chemicals can be detected in the blood, tissues, and fat of humans, sometimes at levels far above "safe" limits. See http://www.panna.org/food-farming-derailed/food-field-fork for more information.

Organically grown food has several advantages over conventionally grown food. A review of 343 publications concludes that organically grown crops contain higher levels of many beneficial compounds, including polyphenols and flavonoids (Baranski et al., 2014). Organic food also contains higher amounts of minerals and vitamins. Organically grown crops contain lower levels of heavy metals like cadmium and have less pesticide residue than conventionally grown food. In some studies, people who eat more organic food have lower rates of obesity and certain types of cancer (Rahman et al., 2024).

If you can only afford to buy some organic food, choose items from the *Dirty Dozen* list, since these foods carry the most chemicals if conventionally grown. You can safely buy conventionally grown items from the *Clean 15* list since they contain less chemical contamination. This list is updated regularly, so go to the EPA website for the most current information.

The Environmental Working Group's Dirty Dozen List		
Strawberries Spinach Kale/collard/mustard greens Peaches	Pears Nectarines Apples Grapes	Bell and hot peppers Cherries Blueberries Green beans
The Environmental Working Group's Clean 15 List		
Avocados Sweet corn Pineapples Onions Papaya	Sweet peas (frozen) Asparagus Honeydew melon Kiwifruit Cabbage	Mushrooms Mangoes Sweet potatoes Watermelon Carrots

Environmental Working Group 2023 Dirty Dozen and Clean 15 Lists

https://www.ewg.org/foodnews/dirty-dozen.php

Avoiding Metabolic Syndrome

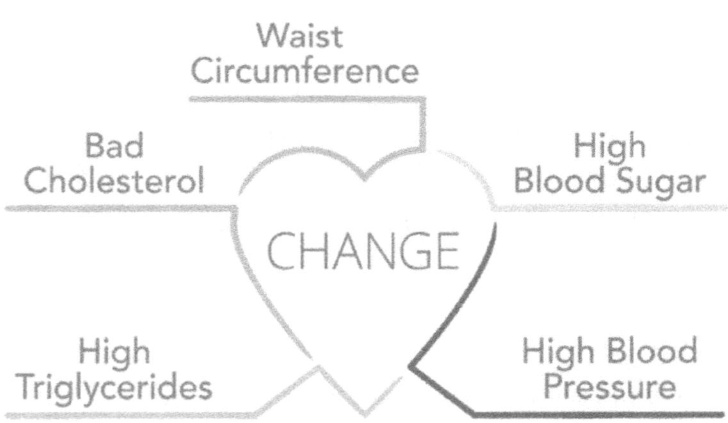

The Five Components of Metabolic Syndrome

Used with permission from Metabolic Syndrome Canada

https://www.metabolicsyndromecanada.ca/mets

It is now widely understood that poor food choices cause metabolic syndrome. Metabolic syndrome, quickly becoming the most expensive and prevalent health problem in developed countries, includes high blood pressure, high waist/hip ratio, high cholesterol, insulin resistance (and diabetes), and heart disease. Metabolic syndrome is implicated in inflammation and chronic disease in general, from autoimmune disorders to Alzheimer's disease. If you want to save your brain, read on.

Metabolic syndrome is caused by eating a high-calorie, high-glycemic diet. Glycemic load refers to how fast the food eaten is broken down into glucose. All foods eventually become sugar. However, protein and fat cause the conversion to work slowly, allowing the body to distribute them slowly and gradually to the tissues. Insulin is the hormone that directs glucose from the bloodstream to the tissues. Complex and simple carbohydrates become sugar quickly and overload the pancreas's ability to make enough insulin.

In a frequent overload situation, the insulin receptors on the tissue cells become less sensitive, the body develops insulin resistance, and this eventually leads to diabetes. Metabolic Syndrome is also associated with inflammation. Inflammation has different outcomes in each organ. Inflammation in the arteries causes heart disease and stroke.

The markers of metabolic syndrome are easily measured. Tests measuring some of these outcomes include fasting blood glucose, fasting serum insulin, cholesterol, triglycerides, apolipoprotein B, and highly sensitive C-reactive protein (Cardiac CRP). These tests are all widely available.

Digestion

Digestion starts in the mouth with the production of amylase, a digestive enzyme in the saliva. It continues with acid production in the stomach and then, with multiple enzymes produced by the pancreas, mixes with the food in the small intestine. Studies suggest that people with chronic illness produce less acidity than healthy people and, as a result, may not digest their food adequately.

Eating more slowly gives the food more time to mix with the enzymes and acid and will aid digestion. Adding the supplement Betaine Hydrochloride (Betaine HCL) at the start of a meal can aid digestion. Although I am not aware of any research to support this clinical observation, many patients with ME/CFS, FM and MCS report feeling better when they add digestive enzymes to their meals. Recommended trials include

Product: Betaine Hydrochloride & Pepsin

Aids in the initial digestion process in the stomach.

Supplier: Thorne Research and others.

Available: Health care professionals and some compounding pharmacies.

Absorption

Inadequate absorption of nutrients may occur in the setting of a *leaky gut*. This is a lay term for the condition in which the intestinal cells lining the gut are unhealthy and cannot maintain the usual tight junctions between cells. These junctions prevent molecules from entering or leaving the body in an uncontrolled manner. People with irritable bowel syndrome (IBS) (common in ME/CFS, FM and MCS) may have leaky gut. In leaky gut, incompletely digested food molecules and bacterial products are able to enter the body.

Building on the work of Dr. Kenny De Meirleir, Dr. Michael Maes and colleagues have shown increased immune reactions in the blood to normal gut bacteria in people with ME/CFS (Maes et al., 2007; Maes & Leunis, 2008). This suggests that the molecules produced by bacteria, which normally live in the colon, are leaking into the body, activating the immune system. Since we know that ME/CFS is a condition associated with immune activation, managing leaky gut may be important. The possibility of poor absorption of needed nutrients and/or loss of nutrients also exists.

How do you tell if you have leaky gut? The gold standard test for leaky gut is the lactulose/mannitol test. It is most easily available through private labs, such as Genova Diagnostics in the US. The treatment for leaky gut encompasses most of the information covered in this session, including avoiding foods to which you are allergic or sensitive, improving the mix of bacteria that live in your colon (more about this under Dysbiosis), and taking supplements to improve the health of the enterocytes and colonocytes (cells that line the small and large bowel). This includes

Product: L-glutamine 500 - 1000 mg up to three times daily.

L-glutamine is the largest concentration of amino acid in the body, which supplies energy to muscle cells as well as to the cells lining the gut. Many people find supplementation with L-glutamine decreases symptoms of leaky gut, such as gas, bloating, and IBS.

Available: Most health food stores.

Food Sensitivities and Allergies

It is very hard to know if a person has sensitivities or allergies to food unless the reaction is immediate and obvious, such as a peanut allergy causing swelling of the throat or itchy hives. Symptoms can occur in any part of the body, including worsening of pain, depression, or cognitive symptoms.

Many allergies are delayed, and many adverse food reactions are not allergic in nature. A non-allergic reaction is not accompanied by an elevation in immune globulin (Ig) levels. In these cases, you may have a food sensitivity or food intolerance. Conventional allergy tests can be negative even in the presence of allergy-related symptoms. This is because conventional tests measure only one type of allergic reaction—those mediated by immunoglobulin E (IgE).

You will see below that I have found the ELISA food allergy blood test clinically useful. Although not 100% accurate (i.e., there can be false positives and false negatives), many patients have been alerted by this test to foods that cause symptoms but that they had never suspected before the test. There is debate about the validity of this test, so, as with all other recommendations in the manual, be aware that little is straightforward in this field.

In my experience, about 50% of patients have identifiable food sensitivities that meet the gold standard test of elimination/reintroduction. If a food allergy or sensitivity exists, the symptoms should go away when the food is eliminated from the diet for a week or more and increase when the food is reintroduced. If one goes through this test three times with the same result, I consider this a valid and more accurate measure than any laboratory test.

There are many touted ways to test for food sensitivities, including blood tests, skin tests, and electrodermal or bioenergetic testing. However, none are as effective as simply eliminating a food from the diet for at least 5 days and then eating it purposely in large enough amounts to challenge the system.

Medical conditions such as celiac disease are also causes of a vast array of gastrointestinal and non-intestinal symptoms. I have missed more than one case of Celiac Disease in people who didn't have diarrhea (the cardinal symptom). Accurate blood testing for Celiac Disease is now easily available through the public health care system and should be ordered in every patient with ME/CFS, FM and MCS.

Scratch testing for food allergies is available through allergists. However, these generally include only a small number of common allergens. And as I've already noted, only IgE allergies will show positive on skin testing. Remember that many food allergies in ME/CFS, FM and MCS are not IgE-mediated. An alternative allergy test to consider is an ELISA panel:

Test: ELISA blood test for IgG + IgE antibodies

Available: Many labs, including Genova and Meridian Labs

Limitations: Only identifies food sensitivities or allergies that are mediated by IgG or IgE. It is prone to false positives and negatives. It is helpful but not a gold standard. The gold standard is the elimination diet with reintroduction of foods.

Elimination Diet

An elimination diet is a method of identifying foods to which a person is sensitive. It is not a long-term eating plan! Here's how it works. All foods are eliminated for 4 days except for one type of meat, one fruit, one vegetable, and one grain. Traditionally, lamb, pears and rice are considered the "safe foods." However, if you know you are sensitive to these, you will need to choose some other foods for the elimination phase. It takes at least 5 days for the other foods and their effects to be eliminated from the system.

After the elimination phase, reintroduce foods one at a time, starting with those you believe are safe. All effects are observed and recorded. Without writing down your observations, you will become hopelessly confused.

If you have an adverse reaction of any kind, eliminate that food and try again after several weeks. If you appear to tolerate a new food, keep it in your diet and eat it every 4-5 days (see rotation diet below). If you eat a tolerated food every day or in large amounts, you risk losing that food. The elimination diet is the best method for identifying food reactions, as it will identify reactions due to allergies or non-allergic "sensitivities." However, this method takes a long time, and many people have difficulty with such a limited diet.

Rotation Diet

Once problem foods have been identified, safe foods should be eaten in a rotation so that the body doesn't become too sensitive to any one food. This is only true for people with food problems. People with no food-related symptoms don't need to follow this advice. Most rotation diets suggest rotating every 4-5 days. In a 4-day rotation, you eat certain foods (or food families) on day one, different foods on day two, yet different foods on day three and yet different foods on day four. Then, repeat the rotation without eating any food or food from the same family more often than every four days. An example rotation diet is included below. It divides food into categories: meat, vegetables, fruit, seeds, nuts, and treats. For example, in the carbohydrate column, potato and potato products are eaten one day, the next rice, the next wheat, the next millet, sweet potato, and so on.

In its purest form, each food should only be eaten once on the day it is allowed. However, the technique still seems to work if each food is eaten throughout the day and then not for at least 4 days. In this way, the body eliminates each food by the time it is eaten again, and if a reaction is present, it will be unmasked and more noticeable.

Symptoms to watch for can be anywhere in the body and can include fatigue, weakness, pain, gastrointestinal or psychological symptoms. Treatment involves the total elimination of identified foods for 6 months and then a re-challenge. If the food is tolerated after a period of abstinence, it should only be eaten in rotation (i.e., not more than every fourth day) to prevent re-sensitization. By keeping to a rotation diet regularly, you can diagnose and treat food sensitivities.

Here is an example of a rotation diet.

Rotation Diet Example Menu							
	Meat	**Vegetable**	**Fruit**	**Carbs**	**Oils**	**Nuts**	**Treats**
Day 1	beef	broccoli	apple	wheat	olive oil	brazils	chocolate
	dairy	green beans	citrus	yeast	canola oil	almonds	rice cookies
			pear	rice			
Day 2	fish	legume	bananas	quinoa	avocado oil	peanuts	carob
		squash families	melon family	oats	flax oil	cashew	soy
Day 3	pork	greens, beets	pineapple	potato	hemp oil	pecans	gelatin treats
			peach	barley	sesame oil	walnuts	
			plum				
Day 4	ostrich	turnips	berries	corn	corn oil	filberts	tapioca
	turkey						
Others	eggs	all other veg	all other fruits	all other grains	all other oil		

Dysbiosis

Biosis refers to the bacterial ecology of the colon. It is normal for the colon to be inhabited by bacteria. In fact, several trillion bacteria of several hundred species live in the human colon to the benefit of all. Each person's colon forms a unique ecosystem for the bacteria living there, depending upon where a person lives, their genetics, and their diet. Research in the field of metabolomics (measuring all the molecules in human urine) shows that 90% of the hundreds of chemical products found in urine are produced not by human cells but by bacteria!

This means that the bacteria growing in the colon have a huge influence on our bodily function. These bugs produce molecules through their normal daily living that are absorbed into our bodies, circulate in the blood, and are excreted in the urine. Some of these molecules can make us ill. For example, tartrazine, a molecule produced by yeast, causes depression. But many of the products made by these bugs are critical to our health since we cannot make them ourselves. These nutrients include the amino acid serine and vitamin K.

One theory about the cause of irritable bowel syndrome (IBS) is that it is associated with bacterial overgrowth—too many bacteria or too many "bad bacteria." Studies have shown that giving 10 days of antibiotics to wipe out all the bacteria in the colon significantly improves IBS symptoms (Pimentel et al., 2003). However, antibiotics kill all the "good bugs" as well as the bad ones and can cause dangerous antibiotic resistance.

Many suggest treating dysbiosis/leaky gut with probiotics instead of antibiotics. Probiotics are cultures of bacteria known to keep the bad bugs in check. Natural bacterial sources, such as yogurt and kefir, are preferred since they have many species of bacteria and are less costly, especially if one is able to grow the cultures on an ongoing basis. For those who are intolerant to milk or soy products, probiotic supplements may be helpful.

Different probiotic species have been shown to be effective for different problems. Therefore, it pays to read up on a product before trying it. I recommend trying different products and rotating products to get the best results. Probiotics only remain in the gut for 7-10 days after ingestion. Therefore, ongoing use is needed unless one is able to change the gut ecology by changing diet or other health factors. There are many different probiotic products, including

Product: VSL#3®

contains a mixture of live freeze-dried lactic acid bacteria, 450 billion bacteria per packet. Research on this product shows benefit in people with severe bowel disorders.

Available: https://www.vsl3.com/ The product will be delivered by courier on ice, as it needs to stay at 4 degrees Celsius.

Product: Fibre Smart®

is flax fibre, probiotic, L-glutamine and other bowel tonics (fennel seed, marshmallow root, slippery elm and others).

Supplier: https://www.renewlife.ca/product/fibresmart-capsules/

Part II. Diagnosis and Treatment of Gastrointestinal Symptoms

Gastrointestinal symptoms are extremely varied in ME/CFS, FM and MCS. Among the most common symptoms are the following:

- Anorexia (loss of appetite)
- Nausea
- Diarrhea

- Constipation
- Abdominal pain

It is very difficult to give guidance as to when the above gastrointestinal symptoms should be a reason for medical consultation. If the symptom is severe enough to cause you discomfort, loss of sleep, poor nutrition, weight loss, or other concerning symptoms, you should consult with your physician.

Anorexia

Anorexia is the medical term for low appetite and does not refer to Anorexia Nervosa, a psychiatric condition marked by the perpetual quest for control and thinness. Anorexia can be associated with any severe medical illness. It is marked in advanced cancer and HIV AIDS. Though not often mentioned as being associated with ME/CFS, FM and MCS, I find it can occur in severely ill individuals, especially with these conditions.

The cause of anorexia in these conditions is unknown. It may be due to a lack of energy of the gastrointestinal system to process food, resulting in a message being sent to the brain not to overload the system with more food. Like nausea, discussed below, anorexia is a very difficult problem because good nutrition is so important to recovery.

Some drugs with increased appetite as a side effect may help, but none have been explicitly studied for this purpose. Examples include: the tricyclic antidepressants such as amitriptyline, the antidepressant mirtazapine, the pain medication pregabalin, and the medical formulations of tetrahydrocannabinol (THC).

Nausea

Nausea is a normal response to toxic substances. Nausea is also associated with low adrenal and thyroid function, as well as other medical conditions. Nausea is common in ME/CFS, FM and MCS and can be disabling. The cause of nausea in ME/CFS, FM and MCS is unclear. Nausea is hard to treat because it is often continuous, whereas most treatments are time-limited and must be repeated. The urge to vomit is influenced by the neurotransmitters: serotonin, dopamine, and endogenous opiates. The commonly used "older" anti-emetics (anti-nausea drugs) include dopamine blockers, such as chlorpromazine and metoclopramide, and antihistamines, such as dimenhydrinate (Gravol®). These are effective for many types of nausea and vomiting, including nausea caused by cancer chemotherapy, but can cause side effects with prolonged use.

Newer antiemetics include drugs that block the serotonin 3 receptors. Ondansetron (Zofran®) is the prototype of this family. Given at a dose of 8 mg approximately 30 minutes before eating, nausea is reduced. Side effects include warm flushing, headaches, and constipation. Ondansetron is very effective but lasts only a few hours.

Diarrhea

Proper diagnosis of the cause of diarrhea is important. Diarrhea with gas and bloating can be caused by many things. If diarrhea is severe, daily, not only associated with food, or is associated with bleeding or weight loss, you should see your doctor. It is likely the doctor will recommend a colonoscopy to rule out various types of colitis.

Diarrhea that is diet-related generally comes on after eating certain foods or slowly gets worse as the day progresses and more foods are eaten. If the diarrhea does not seem food-related, the next step is to rule out an infection. Stool testing for common toxins, such as Clostridium difficile, pathogenic E. coli, and Giardia, is available through most labs. However, these are only a few of the numerous infections that can cause diarrhea.

Diarrhea can also be caused by an overgrowth of bacteria in the usually sterile small bowel, a condition called small bowel bacterial overgrowth or SIBO. The test for this is a hydrogen/methane breath test, which is often hard to access.

Another way to test for bacterial or yeast overgrowth in the gut (colon mostly) is to measure the molecules that these bugs create. These molecules fall into the chemical umbrella of organic acids. Organic acids are molecules formed by biochemical pathways by humans and bugs and are excreted in the urine. If there are high levels of molecules that only bugs produce, this is very strong evidence for overgrowth. Tests for this include the following:

Test: Urinary Organic Acids, Dysbiosis Panel

Available: Mosaic Labs https://mosaicdx.com/test/organic-acids-test/

Test: Quantitative measure of bacterial DNA in the stool

Available: Genova Laboratory or Doctor's Data

- CAUTION must be used with any treatments for diarrhea. If infection is present, drugs to decrease diarrhea can make the infection worse. Undiagnosed colitis is dangerous.
- Bulking agents, such as psyllium (Metamucil®), decrease diarrhea by absorbing water and adding bulk to the stool. This is the most tested and effective treatment for irritable bowel syndrome.

- Cholestyramine (Questran®) decreases diarrhea by binding bile acids and some bacterial toxins. The dose is 4g up to four times per day. Cholestyramine must not be taken with food, drugs, or nutritional supplements, as it will bind to them.
- Loperamide (Imodium®) is 50X stronger than opiates such as morphine in slowing the bowel. Anyone on opiates for pain will have respect for that statistic. Loperamide also increases anal sphincter tone and therefore helps in some cases of fecal incontinence.

Constipation

Constipation can be a difficult and chronic problem, especially for people on certain drugs (e.g., tricyclic antidepressants, opiates). A subset of patients with ME/CFS and FM have congenitally sluggish bowels, and treating this lifelong problem is challenging.

- Any new onset of constipation should be investigated since obstructions due to cancer, adhesions, or inflammatory bowel disease must be ruled out.
- CAUTION must be used with any of the following treatments unless obstruction has been ruled out.
- CAUTION: Many laxatives used over time can cause side effects. They should be used only when needed and should be rotated if possible.
- 20 g/day or more of fibre from diet and added fibre (e.g., psyllium, flax) is widely recommended.
- Osmotic laxatives (e.g., magnesium citrate or sulfate) act by increasing water in the stool and by promoting peristalsis. One dose produces 300-600 mL of stool within 6 hours.
- Lactulose also acts by increasing water in the stool. This is best used before bed at a dose of 15-30 mL. Effects may take 1-2 days of regular use.
- Docusate sodium (Colace®) is a stool emollient; it makes the stool more slippery. Despite widespread use, studies do not show docusate to be very effective.
- Stimulant laxatives (Bisacodyl® and others) are taken at bedtime, 10-15 mg, with an effect expected in the morning. Use for more than 10 days at a time is not recommended, as they can damage the intestinal mucosa.
- Stimulant laxative precursors, such as aloe, cascara, and senna, are activated by bacteria in the colon to make molecules that stimulate colonic contractions. Regular use for 4 months has been associated with discoloration of the colonic mucosa. It is not as serious a condition as was once thought.
- Ellie's remedy for chronic constipation not due to bowel obstruction is the following:
    - Buffered vitamin C: begin at 500 mg three times daily and increase slowly up to 6000 mg per day in divided doses until stools loosen.

- Magnesium supplements (any type): begin at 250 mg three times daily with the vitamin C and increase up to 2000 mg per day in divided doses until stools loosen.
- This combination will work if doses are high enough. Vit C + Mg has other benefits, such as antioxidant activity (vit C) and muscle relaxation (Mg). Some patients have difficulty finding an optimal dose and alternate between constipation and diarrhea.

Abdominal Pain

Abdominal pain has many causes, including irritable bowel syndrome (which is covered in the next section). In general, this pain is divided into two categories. The first, and the one that needs to be ruled out in all patients with abdominal pain, is pain from structural problems, such as a growing cancer or an inflammatory problem, such as Crohn's disease. Bowel cancer in the early stages is painless, noted only in lucky individuals by blood in the stool. It is recommended, therefore, that every person have a screening colonoscopy at age 50 and regularly thereafter to pick up bowel cancers before they are large enough to cause pain and while they are small enough to be treatable. Pain from structural problems is generally constant, present day and night and may or may not be associated with eating and bowel habits.

The other category, functional bowel/abdominal pain, refers to pain not caused by some physical structure or injury, but by problems with the function of the bowel (or other abdominal organ). Irritable Bowel Syndrome, the pain experienced by many with ME/CFS, FM and MCS, is thought to fall into this category. It tends to come and go and is directly related to eating and elimination. There is also abdominal pain unrelated to the bowel, coming from the other organs, muscles or the spine. Only a thorough medical evaluation will be able to distinguish between these types of pain.

Irritable Bowel Syndrome (IBS)

IBS is a chronic pain disorder. The stomach and intestines are especially sensitive to distention. Foods rich in fiber provide food for the bacteria living in the bowel. The bacteria in our colon ferment the food we eat, producing gases such as hydrogen, carbon dioxide and methane. Gas causes distention of the bowel, which in the sensitive IBS bowel leads to pain.

Clinical Presentation

The most common pattern is one of alternating diarrhea and constipation, with one pattern eventually predominating. The diarrhea is often precipitated by emotional stress or eating. Abdominal bloating and flatulence are frequent, as are upper gastrointestinal symptoms, such as nausea and heartburn.

Red flags that some disease other than IBS may be present include weight loss, symptoms at night or first thing in the morning before eating, blood in stool, abnormal physical exam, recent antibiotic use, and family history of colon cancer.

Dietary treatment of IBS

Dietary change is an effective self-management approach to IBS (van Lanen, de Bree, & Greyling, 2021). A group from Monash University in Australia has proposed a diet called the FODMAP diet. FODMAP stands for Fermentable Oligo, Di and Monosaccharides and Polyols. These are all forms of non-absorbable fiber easily fermented by bowel bacteria, resulting in gas production. The gas causes many of the symptoms of IBS, such as bloating, abdominal pain, diarrhea and constipation. Decreasing the intake of these foods results in less fermentation, less gas production and less discomfort.

You can learn more about FODMAPs and the diet at the researchers' website https://www.monashfodmap.com/ibs-central/i-have-ibs/starting-the-low-fodmap-diet/.

Food Group	Low FODMAP Foods to Eat	Foods to Decrease
Fruit	strawberries, oranges, grapes, lemons, limes, bananas, pineapple, and lychee	high fructose fruits like apples, cherries, plums, pears, and watermelon
Vegetables	leafy greens, red bell peppers, spaghetti squash, parsnip, radish, eggplant, bok choy, cucumbers, tomatoes, and mushrooms	artichokes, asparagus, cauliflower, onions, and garlic
Milk	plant-based milks and lactose-free dairy	regular milk, yogurt, and cheese
Proteins	meat, chicken, fish, and eggs are all low FODMAP	soy, beans, tofu, and cashews
Grains	gluten-free grains and traditional sourdough bread	rye, wheat, and barley
Beverages	sweet drinks	best to drink calorie free drinks like water, coffee and tea

FODMAP diet adapted from the website of the Canadian Digestive Health Foundation https://cdhf.ca/en/the-low-fodmap-diet-what-can-i-eat/

Although effective, the FODMAP diet is not recommended for long-term use because it omits too many healthy foods. Fiber is necessary to maintain healthy bacteria in the bowel. It is usually recommended to have a restriction phase followed by the gradual reintroduction of FODMAP-containing foods once the flare-up is past, allowing for a more diverse and healthier long-term diet.

To help people learn and adhere to the diet, the Monash researchers have developed a FODMAP app https://www.monashfodmap.com/get-app-help/.

Drug Treatments for IBS

- Antispasmodics such as dicyclomine (Bentyl®) for patients with abdominal pain.
- Loperamide (Imodium®) for diarrhea (Jailwala et al., 2000).
- If bacterial or fungal overgrowth can be shown, a trial of appropriate anti-infectives is recommended (Nobaek et al., 2000).

Natural Alternatives

- Peppermint oil: decreases muscle spasms, abdominal pain, distention and flatulence. Take 2-4 mg three times daily before meals. Make sure to get an enteric-coated preparation to decrease the side effect of heartburn.
- Probiotics (i.e., good bacteria): when taken regularly for 4 weeks, improve bowel flora (bacterial) balance. Though used by many, it is far from clear that probiotics improve the symptoms of IBS. There is more about probiotics in the section on dysbiosis.
- L-glutamine—this amino acid is one of the preferred foods of the enterocytes (the cells lining the gut: see section on dysbiosis). 500 - 1000mg three times daily is a common dose.

Diet Recommendations

I have learned a lot about diet and diet controversies since this manual was first published. The information in this chapter remains a great foundation. For those wanting to dive deeper into diet, I have an eChapter available online with information on the biology of why diet is so critical to health, the low-carb/low-fat controversy, time-restricted eating, mast cell activation syndrome (MCAS), small intestinal bacterial overgrowth (SIBO) and much more. My new chapters can be found at https://www.eleanorsteinmd.ca/more-light.

Here is a list of my most up-to-date recommendations—a good place to start.

1. **Eat fewer carbohydrates, especially simple sugars and starchy foods.**

   The research evidence is growing that eating fewer carbohydrates is beneficial. A lower-carbohydrate diet benefits cardiovascular health, metabolic syndrome, diabetes and brain health, to name a few conditions. Since medical dogma doesn't change easily, I am sure you will easily find people who disagree with this opinion.

2. **Eat more healthy fat.**

   Naturally occurring fats build healthy cell membranes and maintain hormone production. Most people can benefit from increasing intake of omega-3 fatty acids (EPA and DHA) from small cold-water fish and monounsaturated fatty acids (MUFAs) from olive and avocado oils. Please note this is not a suggestion to eat unhealthy fats from ultra-processed foods.

3. **Eat the rainbow.**

   Colorful, plant-based foods are full of needed nutrients. Eat foods of every color every day, and as many different foods every week as possible.

4. **Time-restricted eating.**

   In consultation with your physician, consider fasting for 12+ hours overnight each 24 hours. This sets the stage for achieving ketosis, if desired, and decreases the risk of dementia through increased disposal of cellular garbage.

5. **Use a continuous glucose monitor** to better understand how your body responds to what you eat.

6. **Identify foods you are sensitive to** and, if you are missing eating them and want to try, gradually reintroduce them through daily neuroplasticity-based practice. Note that successful reintroduction requires adequate preparation of the nervous system and knowledge of appropriate techniques.

7. **Consult a registered dietitian experienced in the area you need help with.**

   If these dietary changes are ineffective in helping you achieve your health goals, seek the assistance of a knowledgeable health care professional. It is easier said than done to find a registered dietitian who has the knowledge needed to assist with these types of diet trials. I would try the "find a clinician" tab on the website of the Institute of Functional Medicine https://www.ifm.org/find-a-practitioner or word of mouth.

Preparing for Session 6

Before reading the next session on toxic load, it is strongly recommended that you spend 2 weeks getting to know and recording chemical and electromagnetic exposures. This will allow you to determine whether chemical or electromagnetic exposures impact your health.

You will need the following:

- A Sleep Chart or an Activity and Symptoms Chart, which you will use to record your reactions to environmental exposures. Joan chose to use the Activity and Symptoms Chart.

Note each time you are exposed to a chemical that you can smell or can't smell but know was present. This includes personal fragrances (yours or other people's), cleaning products, solvents, smells from new furnishings and building products, and petrochemical exhaust—to name just a few. There are over 80,000 man-made or man-altered chemicals in common use, so there is not enough space to list them all.

People are very individual with regard to what types of chemicals may affect them. Even products with natural fragrance, such as essential oils, wood smells, and flowers, can be a problem for some people. Toxic mould is a big problem for many people. Even if the concentration is too low to smell, certain species of mould produce spores and toxins that are hazardous to health.

For identifying electromagnetic exposures, you will need to do some measurements of your home and workplace to see if you are being exposed to higher-than-safe levels of electromagnetic frequency (EMF). You can't see, smell, or feel electricity. There are so many factors to consider that it isn't possible to use a "rule of thumb" to determine if your house is safe or not. You need to measure to know if field levels are high. And you need to observe yourself carefully to determine whether EMF affects your health. Some clues that you might be sensitive to EMF include feeling unwell after talking on the phone or working on the computer for some time.

Useful EMF Measuring Tools

1. High Frequency EMF Analyzer

This allows you to measure frequencies between 800 MHz and 2.5 GHz. This is the frequency range emitted by cell phone towers, cell phones, and wireless technology (e.g., cordless phones, Bluetooth and wireless internet). High-frequency emissions can change moment to moment depending on transmission. The recommended safe limit is below one microWatt/m2. This is the lowest measurable reading on most meters!

2. DC Magnetic Field Analyzer—Liquid Compass

The DC magnetic field is constant and is produced by the Earth itself. Anything that disturbs this natural field can cause symptoms. Disturbances in the Earth's field can be caused by natural sources such as ore deposits and underground water veins or caverns. A disturbance can also be caused by any metal object, including bed frames, cars, magnets in loudspeakers, and phone receivers.

3. AC Magnetic Field/AC and DC Electrical Current Analyzer—TriField Meter

This meter, as you may have guessed, measures three different fields: Alternating Current (AC) Magnetic, AC Electrical (plugged into the wall), and Direct Current (DC) Electrical (battery-powered). Note that this meter will give a qualitative measure, not a digital quantitative readout. Inside the house, AC magnetic fields are produced by all electrical appliances, whether they are AC or DC. Especially problematic are appliances with transformers (e.g., halogen lamps) or AC/DC converters (e.g., answering machines).

Outside the house, an AC magnetic field is produced by power lines. Underground power lines are partially shielded by the earth. If a house is properly wired, magnetic fields caused by circuitry should cancel each other out and be below three milligauss when using the "Magnetic 0-3 range" scale on the TriField Meter. Magnetic current can run along improperly grounded wires, metal pipes, and heating ducts.

4. Body Voltage Analyzer—amp/volt/ohm Meter

This meter can measure many things. In the experiment I will outline, it is used to measure the amount of electrical current that is passing through your body.

Take readings in the key areas of your house, such as the head of your bed, a favourite reading chair, your computer desk, and your sofa. Then have an assistant go to the electrical panel and turn off the power to the house at the electrical panel. Repeat the reading. A safe reading is under 100 mV. Now have your assistant systematically turn on each circuit, beginning with the "essentials." These include the power to the furnace, air ventilation system, fridge, and freezers. Then, turn on one by one the other circuits and identify which electrical circuits are causing hot spots in key areas of the house.

A range of testing equipment is available for loan from my office. Most electricians will possess the equipment necessary, but electricians are generally not aware of the health effects of electricity on sensitive individuals. For more information on dirty electricity, go to:
https://emfacademy.com/dirty-electricity-filter-guide/.

Joan's Activity and Symptoms Chart

Below is Joan's charting for environmental exposures using the Activity and Symptoms Chart. She only wrote down things that she noticed. Some days, she didn't detect any chemical or EMF reactions.

Name: Joan Smith **Date** Jan 30/12 **to** Feb 12/12

Activity and Symptom Chart

Date & Time	Activity	Symptom
Jan 30/12	work	headache 5/10 cause?
every day	walk dog	sore, throbbing ankle, worse if stand or walk 3/10 - 5/10
Feb 2	work boss's cologne?	headache 4/10 felt ill
Feb 4	dinner out	bowel cramps 5/10 most of the night ? garlic
Feb 6	work	felt OK! boss away
Feb 7	father health crisis	muscle pain ↑ 7/10 very worried
Feb 8	rested all day bad sleep	muscle pain still bad 6/10
Feb 9	work (wore mask)	no headache but people stare at me!
Feb 10	grocery shopping	some bowel pain + queasy stomach
Feb 11	bad sleep	↑ muscle pain
Feb 12	church! perfume musty in basement	headache have to wear mask and talk to minister about "no scent" policy.

Session 5 References

Baranski, M., Srednicka-Tober, D., Volakakis, N., Seal, C., Sanderson, R., Stewart, G. B., . . . Leifert, C. (2014). Higher antioxidant and lower cadmium concentrations and lower incidence of pesticide residues in organically grown crops: a systematic literature review and meta-analyses. *British Journal of Nutrition, 112*(5), 794–811. doi:https://dx.doi.org/10.1017/S0007114514001366

Drossman, D.A. (1999). The Rome criteria process: diagnosis and legitimization of irritable bowel syndrome. *Am J Gastroenterol.*, 94, 2803-2807.

Dunstan, R.H., McGregor, N.R., Butt, H., Roberts, T.K., Klineberg, I.J., Niblett, S.H., Rothkirch, T., & Buttfield, I. (2000). Characterisation of differential amino acid homeostasis amongst population subgroups: a basis for determining specific amino acid requirements. *Journal of Nutritional and Environmental Medicine.*

Jailwala, J., Imperiale, T.F., & Kroenke, K. (2000). Pharmacologic treatment of the irritable bowel syndrome: a systematic review of randomized, controlled trials. *Ann.Intern.Med.*, 133, 136-147.

Maes, M. & Leunis, J.C. (2008). Normalization of leaky gut in chronic fatigue syndrome (CFS) is accompanied by a clinical improvement: effects of age, duration of illness and the translocation of LPS from gram-negative bacteria. *Neuro.Endocrinol.Lett.*, 29, 902-910.

Maes, M., Mihaylova, I., & Leunis, J.C. (2007). Increased serum IgA and IgM against LPS of enterobacteria in chronic fatigue syndrome (CFS): indication for the involvement of gram-negative enterobacteria in the etiology of CFS and for the presence of an increased gut-intestinal permeability. *J.Affect. Disord.*, 99, 237-240.

Nobaek, S., Johansson, M.L., Molin, G., Ahrne, S., & Jeppsson, B. (2000). Alteration of intestinal microflora is associated with reduction in abdominal bloating and pain in patients with irritable bowel syndrome. *American Journal of Gastroenterology*, 95, 1231-1238.

Parlor, M. (2009). Profile and impact of 23 chronic conditions in the 2005 Canadian community health survey. *National ME/FM Action Network.*

Pimentel, M., Chow, E.J., & Lin, H.C. (2000). Eradication of small intestinal bacterial overgrowth reduces symptoms of irritable bowel syndrome. *Am J Gastroenterol.*, 95, 3503-3506.

Pimentel, M., Chow, E.J., & Lin, H.C. (2003). Normalization of lactulose breath testing correlates with symptom improvement in irritable bowel syndrome: a double-blind, randomized, placebo-controlled study. *The American Journal of Gastroenterology*, 98, 412-419.

Rahman, A., Baharlouei, P., Koh, E. H. Y., Pirvu, D. G., Rehmani, R., Arcos, M., & Puri, S. (2024). A Comprehensive Analysis of Organic Food: Evaluating Nutritional Value and Impact on Human Health. *Foods (Basel, Switzerland), 13*(2). doi:https://www.mdpi.com/2304-8158/13/2/208

Worthington, V. (2001). Nutritional quality of organic versus conventional fruits, vegetables, and grains. *J Altern.Complement Med.*, 7, 161-173.

Session 6

Lowering the Toxic Load

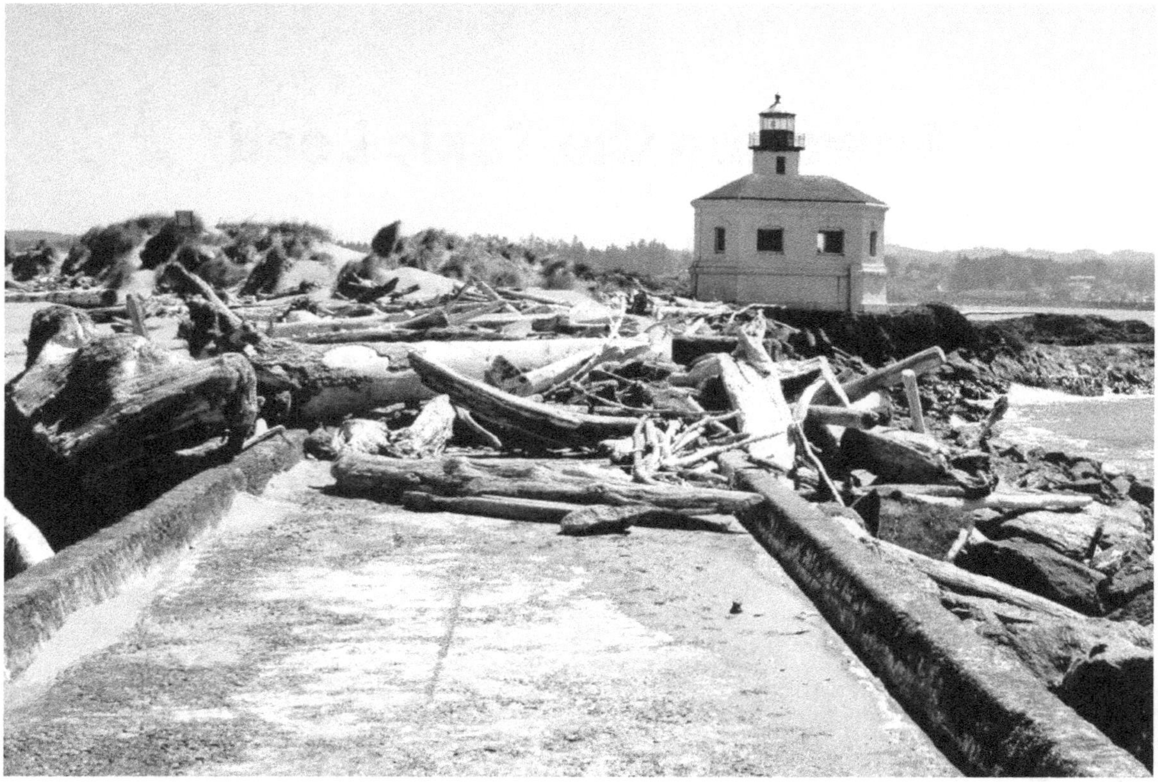

Getting There

We are still on the path.
Our symptoms are more manageable now.
The seemingly unreachable target of wellness is slowly getting closer.
Management is the key.
There are big roadblocks still to be surmounted.
We can do it!
We MUST do it.
We see things clearer now.
Our trials and travels are making sense now.
We CAN do it!

The Road Well Travelled Part III

Session 6

Lowering the Toxic Load

Objectives

- To understand the presentation of Multiple Chemical Sensitivity (MCS).
- To increase knowledge about common toxic exposures inside and outside of the home.
- To learn to track reactions (if any) to toxic exposures.
- To learn strategies to lower toxic load.
- To understand the presentation of Electromagnetic Hyper-Sensitivity (EHS), a newly emerging disorder.

Multiple Chemical Sensitivity

Environmental sensitivity is a common health problem, thought to exist in as many as 15% of the general population (Caress & Steinemann, 2004). Environmental sensitivity is the development of symptoms when exposed to low concentrations of common chemicals that don't affect most people. Now, with increasing awareness of the effects of electromagnetic frequency, the term Environmental sensitivity has expanded to include symptoms caused by both chemicals and electromagnetic frequency. The latter is often referred to as electromagnetic hypersensitivity or EHS.

In severe cases, people with environmental sensitivity meet the case definition for Multiple Chemical Sensitivity or MCS. As many as 40% of patients with ME/CFS and FM also meet criteria for MCS (Lavergne et al., 2010; Bell et al., 1998; Brown & Jason, 2007; Jason et al., 2000). The precise mechanisms for MCS are not yet known. In the absence of knowledge, debate continues about the validity and nature of MCS.

Some physicians continue to believe that MCS is non-existent, is a form of anxiety or is a psychosomatic disorder. However, more than half of the over 500 peer-reviewed medical articles on MCS support an organic basis for MCS. Less than one-quarter support a psychiatric basis (Donnay, 1999). This is not to say that MCS doesn't involve psychological symptoms in many patients (indeed, many conditions involve such symptoms), but the primary triggers appear to be environmental toxins.

For a review of MCS, including references to the varied research about the causes and mechanisms of disease, I recommend the *Environmental Sensitivities-Multiple Chemical Sensitivity Status Report* written by the physicians of the Environmental Health Clinic at Women's College Hospital in Toronto (Marshall, Bested, J., Kerr, & Bray, 2011). Two other excellent Canadian documents are *The Medical Perspective on Environmental Sensitivities* (Sears, 2007) and *Accommodation for Environmental Sensitivities: Legal Perspective* (Wilkie & Baker, 2008), both written for the Canadian Human Rights Commission. The full text can be found on the Government of Canada website, as noted in the citations.

1999 Case Definition of Multiple Chemical Sensitivity

An international consensus process has defined the following clinical profile as necessary for diagnosis (1999):

- MCS is a chronic condition.
- Symptoms recur reproducibly in response to low levels of exposure.
- Symptoms occur in response to multiple unrelated chemicals.
- Symptoms improve or resolve when incitants are removed.
- Symptoms occur in multiple organ systems.
- No other single organ disorder can account for the symptoms.

The 1999 case definition has been validated by a team at the University of Toronto (McKeown-Eyssen et al., 2001). They suggest that some additional symptoms strengthen the discriminant validity of the case definition (the ability to differentiate between people with MCS and other conditions):

- Having a stronger sense of smell than most people.
- Feeling spacey.
- Feeling dull or groggy.
- Having difficulty concentrating.

Consensus documents and position papers on MCS have also been published by the following:

- American Lung Association
- American Medical Association
- U.S. Environmental Protection Agency (EPA)
- U.S. Consumer Product Safety Commission (USCPSC)

What Causes MCS?

The current definition of MCS doesn't fit well with existing linear medical disease models. Patients can become ill from unrelated chemical structures and experience symptoms in different body systems from the same chemical exposure. Modern medicine validates conditions with one cause and one effect. This raises the question: How can we explain the symptom patterns experienced by patients with MCS? Dr. William Rea is a leading environmental physician and the author of an authoritative

4-volume book on the topic *Chemical Sensitivity* (Rea, 1997). In the diagram below from Rea's textbook, the linear models of Virchow and Newton, in which one cause leads to one effect, are compared with the nonlinear model of Pischinger and Heine (Pischinger, 2007). In this model, more than one cause can lead to more than one effect.

Rea also introduces the metaphor of the body as a barrel to help understand some of the puzzling aspects of the illness. Why, for example, does a certain exposure cause minimal symptoms one day and severe symptoms on another day? In this model, as we are exposed to pollutants (and I would add other physical and psychological stressors), the metaphorical barrel fills. While it fills, we are symptom-free. When the barrel overflows, the body's reserve capacity to manage stressors is exhausted, and symptoms result. On some days, the barrel is fuller than others, and it takes less time/exposure for it to overflow.

The main treatment objective in this environmental medicine model of MCS is to decrease the body burden of toxins, sometimes referred to as the *toxic load*. This means preventing the barrel from filling (avoidance) and helping it empty (detoxification and excretion). Not all toxins are man-made; the toxins produced by some mould species create classic symptoms of MCS. MCS is unique among medical conditions in that it does not have a consistent pattern of symptoms or signs, but the pattern of occurrence of symptoms in relation to exposure(s) is typical.

There are many theories about the cause of MCS. The following hypothesis, developed by European researchers, is one of the leading contenders. The body is kept in homeostasis by the ground regulation system (GRS), consisting of end vascular pathways, connective tissue cells, extracellular matrix and nerve endings. This system comprises many of the cells and the *non-cellular matrix* in between the body's organs. The matrix can sometimes be seen as a white, web-like material between organs, but the cellular components are only visible with a microscope.

This matrix is the key to maintaining homeostasis. Homeostasis (keeping the body ecology in balance) relies on speedy and accurate communication between all parts of the body at all times. If the total body load of toxins is too high, balance will be impaired, and symptoms will occur with very little provocation. The GRS is also sensitive to chemical toxins and changes in pH (acid/base balance), electromagnetic currents, and barometric pressure.

The GRS controls oxygen flow, mitochondrial function, and free radical formation. Each of these is critical for each cell to function. Oxygen and glucose (blood sugar) provide the fuel that the mitochondria (small engines of each cell) turn into energy. Free radical molecules are produced because of the burning of oxygen and are damaging to cells. The body's natural antioxidants, such as glutathione, limit this damage. This model explains why many of the symptoms of MCS do not follow nerve anatomy and why symptoms fluctuate frequently. The GRS model may explain the sensitivity of people with MCS to apparently unrelated triggers such as weather changes, electricity, and altitude.

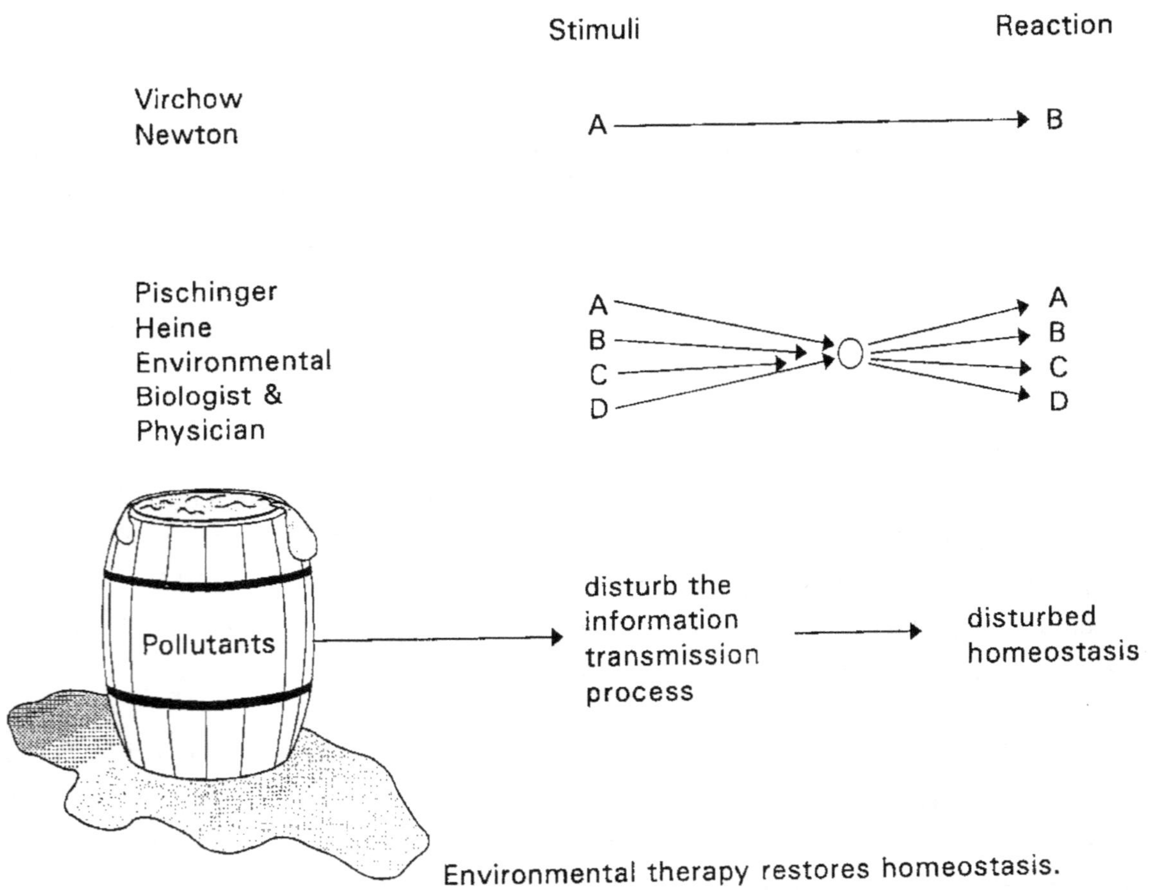

Figure 9. The causes of and therapy for the chemically sensitive patient are based on multi-dimensional function association. Biological systems do not show linearity, but are highly integrated and are subject to biological flow equilibrium.

This diagram from page 2027 of Dr. Rea's 4-volume textbook *Chemical Sensitivity* used with permission from the author.

Some Research Findings in MCS

- Elderly subjects with food intolerance show objectively poorer sleep EEG and different EEG patterns than are found in depression, pesticide poisoning, and insomnia of unknown origin (Bell et al., 1996).
- Women with chemical sensitivity show EEG sensitization when exposed intermittently to chemicals, a reaction not found in women with no history of chemical sensitivity (Fernandez et al., 1999).
- SPECT scans done using the protocol of radiologist, Dr. Theodore Rubin, who works with Dr. Rea, show characteristic changes which are thought to reflect altered glutathione distribution to the brain, and clearance from the brain. Glutathione is one of the body's most important antioxidant molecules.
- Patients with MCS are found to have unfavourable variations in the DNA for some of the genes which control the enzymes of liver metabolism (McKeown-Eyssen et al., 2004).
- Another study reports genetic variation in the genes that control Redox, the state of oxidation and reduction in cells (DeLuca C. et al., 2010).

In 1995, MCS researcher Dr. Claudia Miller conducted a study, now a classic, in which patients who became ill due to pesticide exposure were compared to those who became ill after house remodeling. The patients in the two groups had virtually identical symptoms, even though the offending chemicals were different. As you read the following list of symptoms commonly reported by those with MCS, you may note that these symptoms sound very similar to those of ME/CFS and FM. This has led many to consider the idea that ME/CFS and FM are, in part, caused or triggered by exposure to environmental toxins.

The number of toxins in our environment has markedly increased since World War II, and these toxins are now found in all of us, even those who are healthy. And more concerning, even children are affected. For information on the impact of chemical toxins on the health of children, see the Canadian Partnership for Children's Health and the Environment website at www.healthyenvironmentforkids.ca. For more information on the health impacts of environmental pollutants on humans in general, there are several references at the Ontario College of Family Physicians website: http://www.ocfp.on.ca/committees/env-health.

Below are common symptoms experienced by patients with MCS, according to Miller's research.

Common Symptoms of MCS

(Miller & Mitzel, 1995)

- Tired or lethargic
- Fatigue >6 months
- Memory difficulties
- Difficulty concentrating
- Dizziness, lightheadedness
- Depressed feelings
- Spacey or groggy
- Loss of motivation
- Tense, nervous
- Short of breath
- Irritable
- Problem focusing eyes
- Chest pain
- Muscle aches
- Problems digesting food
- Joint pain
- Tingling fingers/toes

Triggers (include but are not limited to)

- Gasoline, kerosene, natural gas
- Pesticides (especially chlordane and chlorpyrifos)
- Solvents
- New carpet and other renovation materials
- Adhesives/glues
- Fiberglass
- Carbonless copy paper
- Fabric softener
- Formaldehyde and glutaraldehyde
- Carpet shampoos (lauryl sulfate) and other cleaning agents
- Isocyanates (paint hardeners)
- Combustion products (poorly vented gas heaters, overheated batteries)
- Medications including anesthetics

Joan's Activity and Symptoms Chart for Environmental Sensitivities

Look at Joan's Activity and Symptoms Chart and at your own. Before doing this exercise, Joan had been unaware that she was sensitive to anything in particular. She thought that all her symptoms were due to FM or ME/CFS. She suspects now that this is not the case. Now she is going through her house, checking on her reactions to all her cleaning and personal care products. She has done some reading about electromagnetic frequencies (EMFs) and their effect on health, and she plans to hire an electrician to help her measure the Electromagnetic Frequency (EMF) in her house.

What does your chart show? Have you looked through your personal care products? Do any of them contain ingredients with names you can't pronounce, or do they have a skull and crossbones on the label? Are any of them safe enough to drink? If not, why would you put them on your skin or breathe their fumes? Once you have finished the reading below, you might also consider finding out about the EMFs in your environment.

Treatment of MCS: The Environmental Medicine Approach

The goal of environmental medicine is to keep the body's metaphorical barrel well below overflowing. In this state, the body has a reserve to cope with unexpected or unusually high exposures without symptoms developing. A cornerstone in decreasing toxic load is to avoid further exposures. In our polluted world, absolute avoidance is impossible. Pollutants have spread to every niche of our planet; even living in a remote area, eating organic food, drinking filtered water, and breathing filtered air does not guarantee total avoidance. There are several excellent guides to non-toxic products online.

Avoidance of Airborne Toxins

Outdoor air quality: Air quality differs significantly among locations. Try to live and work upwind from polluting industry and built-up areas. Highly sensitive people will have to choose their locations very carefully.

If you are allergic or sensitive to pollens or terpenes (natural smells from trees), ensure you have an airtight house with an excellent ventilation/filter system for the high allergen times of year.

Indoor air quality: In your own residence, it makes sense to avoid the use of all chemicals where possible. Our society is obsessed with cleanliness and decreasing workload. It is possible to have a clean, safe residence without using any products bearing the skull and crossbones logo on the packaging. Cleaning products that are free of fragrance and phosphates, such as the Canadian brand NatureClean®, can substitute for conventional cleaners.

- Hydrogen peroxide can be used as a household disinfectant. Vinegar and water can be used as an all-purpose cleaner. Baking soda can be used to scrub pots and sinks, and borax can be used as a laundry whitener. The internet abounds with recipes for safe and eco-friendly cleaners.
- It is usually possible and affordable to create an oasis in one room to which you may retreat when needed. Ideally, this would be the bedroom, as this is the room where people spend the most time.

- A HEPA and charcoal filter running continuously will decrease particulates, volatile organic compounds, and infective molecules in the oasis room. If you use a HEPA filter, make sure to read the specifications to ensure it will clean the size of the area you have in mind and will filter out the compounds you want. Make sure that you vacuum the pre- and post-carbon filters and replace the HEPA filters when you notice they aren't working anymore. These filters actually fill up with particles and chemical fumes, and at a certain point, they just can't absorb any more.
- Humidifiers should not be used as they are breeding spots for mould and bacteria.
- The oasis room should be carefully checked for water damage (e.g., discoloration of walls, buckling ceilings or flooring). Water damage allows mould to grow.
- Hardwood or ceramic flooring releases much fewer toxins than carpets or soft linoleum.
- Furniture should be made of natural materials (e.g., wood or metal) to minimize off-gassing chemicals found in particleboard and epoxy glue. The paint should be free of volatile organic compounds (VOCs) or be well off-gassed.
- No scented products should be kept in the bedroom (e.g., scented candles, incense, and air fresheners). Clothing worn in the outside world should not be brought into the bedroom.
- Mattresses should be made of natural materials and not contain fungicides, antibacterials or fire-retardant chemicals. They should be covered with a dense fibre cover so that dust mites do not accumulate. Bedding should be organic, natural fibre and washed frequently in fragrance-free, non-toxic detergent. Sunlight kills infectives naturally through ultraviolet light, so ensure that the room is aired and receives direct sunlight.

When you can't avoid toxic exposures: One of the most isolating aspects of having MCS is that most public places are filled with chemicals. Stores, for example, have chemicals off-gassing from products they sell, cleaners, printers, building materials, and employees and customers. Although you will get a lot of stares, many patients successfully use face masks to limit exposure. Surgical masks (the blue ones many people wear when ill or trying to avoid infection) do not work for volatile organic compounds, which comprise the majority of toxins you will come into contact with. For this purpose, one needs a mask with a carbon filter.

Many patients use Respro® brand masks or similar brands with removable filters that can be replaced as needed. Sometimes they are sold at cycling stores, as many cyclists and bike couriers use them to avoid breathing in exhaust. https://respro.com/pollution-masks

Avoidance of Water-Borne Toxins

Water should be filtered to eliminate chlorine, heavy metals, and other chemicals such as medications and pesticides. These chemicals are so widely used that they have leached into virtually all water supplies. Active filtering is preferable to buying bottled water that is stored in plastic containers. Plastic contains phthalates and other toxins, which leach into the water. Ask for the test results on any filter you are considering buying to ensure it addresses a wide range of toxins as well as infectious agents.

Avoidance of Food-Borne Toxins

Conventional food contains measurable amounts of hormones, antibiotics, herbicides, and pesticides, as well as preservatives and chemicals to enhance color, texture, etc. These chemicals can be detected in the blood, tissues, and fat of humans, sometimes at levels far above "safe" limits. See http://www.panna.org/issues/food-agriculture/pesticides-on-food for more information. Organic food contains more nutritional content than conventionally grown food (Worthington, 2001). Avoid processed food, and if your budget allows, buy organic food.

Sauna Therapy

Sauna is the most well-studied method of detoxification. Saunas facilitate the excretion of fat-soluble toxins such as DDE (a byproduct of the pesticide DDT) and PCBs. It has been shown that sauna therapy causes a measurable reduction in the body burden of these chemicals (Genuis et al., 2011; Rea, 1997). Ongoing use of a sauna decreases sympathetic stimulation and cardiovascular responses (51% improved, 9% worse and 40% unchanged in a study of 1000 patients at the EHC Dallas).

Dry saunas are preferred over wet ones since they are less difficult to keep clean. Wet saunas and steam rooms tend to attract mould growth. Infrared saunas are very popular and are being sold as a better choice than other types of saunas (e.g., ceramic or electric heat). I have not read any reliable, independent data confirming the benefits of infrared saunas compared with other types. In my opinion, any dry sauna that reliably causes sweating will be helpful for detoxification. For those who are able, vigorous exercise causing sweating is also excellent for detoxification. Here are some pointers when using sauna therapy:

- Sauna detoxification must be done slowly to avoid mobilization of more toxins than the body can handle.
- Some protocols suggest starting as low as 120 degrees Fahrenheit, some start at 160 degrees, which is the temperature that most people eventually use.
- A typical time in a sauna is 40 minutes.

- Sauna can be used as tolerated (up to once daily).
- Use of a sauna should be accompanied by use of supplemental minerals and amino acids, since these are lost or used up with detoxification.
- Exercise also aids in detoxification; therefore, it is good to take a sauna after exercise (as tolerated).

Sauna Really Does Work.
The evidence for sauna therapy in detoxification continues to build. Dr. Stephen Genuis and colleagues have found that sauna results in excretion of heavy metals, phthalates and polychlorinated biphenyls such as BPA in sweat (S.J. Genuis, Beesoon, Birkholz, & Lobo, 2012; Stephen J. Genuis, Beesoon, Lobo, & Birkholz, 2012; S.J. Genuis, Birkholz, Rodushkin, & Beesoon, 2011).

A paper from Australia systematically reviews the medical literature on the potential benefits of dry sauna therapy (far infrared and plain heat) and finds evidence of benefit for many health conditions, including FM and ME/CFS (Hussain & Cohen, 2018). Sauna is surprisingly well-tolerated except in the study of ME/CFS, in which patients reported intolerance of the heat. In my practice, even people who are sensitive to heat on hot summer days tolerate sauna well.

As with any other therapy, sauna should be undertaken with the awareness of a knowledgeable health professional. There are protocols to maintain safety, prevent dehydration, replace minerals lost in sweat and prevent toxins from being reabsorbed. By working with a health care professional, you can access this information and optimize the impact of sauna.

In addition to aiding detoxification, sauna is now known to be a beneficial stressor, triggering the body's innate healing capacity. Regular sauna use of 20 minutes/session is associated with reduced morbidity and mortality. The biological effects are similar to those resulting from physical exercise. Sauna improves heart rate variability (parasympathetic tone) and cardiovascular health. It has generalized anti-inflammatory effects, decreases oxidative stress and even increases brain-derived neurotropic factor, resulting in improved brain health (Patrick & Johnson, 2021). In my experience, it takes longer than 20 minutes to heat up and get a really good sweat going. I generally sauna for 30 – 40 minutes.

Cholestyramine

- Cholestyramine is a prescription drug that has been used for many decades for the treatment of high cholesterol. It acts by binding to cholesterol and other fat-soluble toxins in the bowel and not allowing them to be reabsorbed.
- Cholestyramine also aids in the removal of fat-soluble toxins, including mould-produced toxins and man-made toxins from the body (Genuis et al., 2010; Shoemaker & House, 2006).

- The recommended dose is one pkg or 4g up to four times daily, 2 hours after and 30 minutes before eating. This protocol is very difficult to follow. Like a sauna, I would say it's better to use some cholestyramine regularly than not at all. It allows excretion of toxins that cannot be removed by any other method.
- Cholestyramine is not absorbed and is therefore a very safe drug; it does, however, cause constipation and should be taken with fibre and fluids.
- If you want to try Cholestyramine, you will need to discuss this with your doctor. If your cholesterol levels are very low, as is the case with some severely ill patients, you should not use this drug.

Rebuilding a Healthy Body

In conventional medicine, nutritional supplements are used to stave off disease (e.g., eat oranges to prevent scurvy). In functional medicine, the goal is to assist the body to function as well as possible, not merely to avoid illness. This goal of optimal health rests on a bedrock of a healthy diet and often includes using supplements to optimize cellular function. As discussed in Session 5, I recommend testing of nutrient levels and function rather than assuming supplements are needed. If you compare the cost of the test against the cost of buying years' worth of unneeded supplements, you may choose the former. (Much of this was covered in Session 5, but since it is such an important part of the whole Environmental Medicine approach, it is repeated here.)

- Avoid foods that make your symptoms worse (rotation diet).
- Eat a nutritionally dense diet (outer aisles of the supermarket).
- Consider a trial of digestive enzymes/betaine HCl if you think you might not be digesting your food well. Digestive enzymes increase the amount of food that is fully digested. Betaine HCl replaces hydrochloric acid in the stomach. As I mentioned in Session 5, this is often deficient in people with chronic illness.
- Vitamin and mineral supplementation can help ensure that cell enzymes can work properly.
- Amino acid supplementation may assist with protein building and liver detoxification.
- Fatty acid supplementation—replaces "bad fat" in the cell membranes and improves cell function.

Mast Cell Activation Syndrome (MCAS)

An emerging hypothesis about the causation of MCS is a condition called Mast Cell Activation Syndrome (MCAS). This condition has been described in the medical literature for less than a decade (a nanosecond in the timeline of medical research), and solid supporting research is lacking. However, the similarities between MCAS and MCS are striking, and MCAS could be a contributor.

Mast cells are immune cells found in tissues that interact with the external environment—tissues such as the gut, lungs and skin. The job of mast cells is to protect the body against invaders. People with seasonal allergies, asthma and peanut allergy are very familiar with the effects of histamine release.

People with MCAS are thought to have highly sensitive mast cells, which are triggered to release their immune chemical contents in response to things like foods, medication, heat, stress and other things that most people aren't allergic to. When this chemical soup is released, the number and variety of ensuing symptoms are huge. As you read the list of MCAS symptoms below, you will note the overlap in the symptoms of MCAS with all of ME/CFS, FM and MCS.

Typical Mast Cell Activation Signs and Symptoms (note these are a few of the most common symptoms from a very long and varied list—different authors have different lists)

- Feeling unwell forever—fatigue and malaise are common
- Abdominal pain and tenderness, nausea, diarrhea and bloating, especially after eating
- Episodic symptoms like flushing, itching, and sweating that wax and wane
- Rashes that come and go, including hives and angioedema
- Heart palpitations, fast heart rate and dizziness
- Brain fog and headache

Triggers include heat, stress, exercise, alcohol, insect bites, drugs such as NSAIDS (anti-inflammatories), antibiotics and opiates and chemical exposures such as to perfume, cleaning products and smoke.

Diagnosis

- Typical symptoms from the above list in at least two body systems.
- Elevation in a mast cell mediator, such as serum alpha-tryptase, above baseline on lab testing.
- More than 50% reduction in symptoms with drugs that block the production or activity of mast cells.

Features of Mast Cell Activation
adapted from papers by Dr. Matthew Hamilton (Hamilton, 2018) and
Peter Valent (Valent et al., 2019)

Since I learned about and started looking for MCAS, I identified many patients who meet the criteria and whose symptoms are at least in part controlled by antihistamines. It is possible that mast cell activation is an underlying cause for a subgroup of individuals who are diagnosed with ME/CFS, FM or MCS. I especially suspect MCAS in patients who have episodic symptoms as outlined in response to foods, supplements, drugs and toxins and who have histamine-related symptoms such as hives, itching and explosive bowel symptoms.

There are many drugs that can be helpful, and improvement with drug therapy supports diagnosis. Among the most used symptomatic drug remedies are antihistamines (H1 and H2 blockers), drugs used in different allergic conditions such as cromolyn sodium, ketotifen, montelukast and supplements such as quercetin and luteolin.

To learn more about this complex disorder, I recommend the website of the Mast Cell Disease Society www.tmsforacure.org/.

The Mind-Body Hypothesis

Many people develop MCS after exposure to known toxins. Many others are exposed to toxins and do not develop chronic sensitivity. People with MCS become more and more sensitive to lower concentrations of toxic molecules. This transformation may be due to a normal, protective brain process called central sensitization. If the brain records that a certain trigger is dangerous, to keep us safe, it may continue to let us know when we are exposed to even tiny amounts of that molecule or even experiences that are similar to the exposure incident. Central sensitization (CS) is defined as "a hyper excitement of the central neurons through various synaptic and neurotransmitter/ neurochemical activities" (Yunus 2007).

Conditions influenced by CS share common symptoms such as pain, fatigue, poor sleep, and sensitivity to noxious and non-noxious stimuli, ultimately impacting health-related quality of life. CS perpetuates and strengthens these debilitating symptoms; downregulating CS may result in improved quality of life.

Increasingly, people are having success with mind-body interventions (MBIs) that harness the complex interaction between mind and body to improve health and well-being. The brain is constantly recording our lived experiences, and we can get caught in a cycle of triggers, symptoms, fear and avoidance in which the brain generates more and more symptoms to get our attention and keep us safe. Sometimes there is no danger, but the brain didn't get the memo. It keeps generating symptoms long after the danger has passed.

MBIs teach consistent, self-directed use of purposeful thoughts, feelings and actions that support changes in biology and function. There is fMRI evidence that practicing MBIs changes brain structure and function (Gotink, 2016). There is an increasing number of small studies suggesting this mind-body approach may be effective for symptoms of complex chronic conditions, although MCS has not been specifically studied. In my experience over the past 10 years, MCS can respond well to this approach. I have fully recovered from MCS using mind-body strategies.

The core strategies of effective mind-body approaches include calming the nervous system and developing a lived sense of safety. This requires reframing the amount of danger from ongoing exposures. Repeatedly redirecting attention away from symptoms, triggers, and negative emotions towards fun, creativity, and connection helps rewire neural circuits to generate comfort and vitality rather than symptoms. Slowly increasing normal life activities show the brain, through lived experience, that we are safe. For many people, starting with imaginary exposure is a good first step, moving to real exposure as you gain capacity and confidence. I have developed two courses teaching these strategies. You can find more information on my website at https://www.eleanorsteinmd.ca/courses.

An important note: Randomized controlled trials are needed to see whether these mind-body approaches are effective. If they are not, people need to know so they can stop spending money on treatments that don't work. If research confirms that mind-body approaches are effective for MCS, hopefully, they will move into the mainstream so that all people with MCS can access training.

Regardless, I advocate minimizing exposure to toxins. Man-made toxins are bad for health, and we cannot build tolerance. Preventive management of toxic exposures through the many strategies discussed in this session is prudent.

Electrohypersensitivity

In 2005, Electromagnetic Hypersensitivity (EHS) was defined by the World Health Organization as “a phenomenon where individuals experience ill effects when in the vicinity of devices emanating electrical, magnetic, or electromagnetic fields.”
See http://www.who.int/mediacentre/factsheets/fs296/en/index.html for the WHO fact sheet on EHS.

The universal presence of electromagnetic waves in our living, working, and playing spaces is suspected of causing health problems. This is because human cells and human bodies are electromagnetic organisms. Man-made electricity and radiofrequency waves have the capacity to interfere with normal cellular functioning.

The two major types of Electromagnetic Frequency (EMF) include the very low frequencies emitted by electrical wiring, appliances, and power lines, and the much higher frequency radiation emitted by radio and wireless devices (Parsons, 2007). In addition, you may have heard about stray or “dirty electricity" formed when different currents interact with each other, forming new frequencies referred to as harmonics. This is thought to have ill effects as well (Havas, 2006).

The BioInitiative Report

BioInitiative is a non-profit group of international scientists who read and summarize the world literature on the effects of electromagnetic radiation on living organisms. They wrote a comprehensive report in 2007. It was updated in 2012, and a lay summary was published in 2014. The 2012 report reviewed over 1800 studies published since 2007 and concluded that the EMF causes a wide range of adverse health effects. More recent updates on several sections of the report are available on the BioInitiative website www.bioinitiative.org/.

The reports explain why most national safety standards, including Canada's regarding EMF exposure, are not safe. Existing safety standards rely on the assumption that damage from EMF occurs only through the heat produced by high-frequency EMF. However, the report notes that this is incorrect. Damage occurs at exposure levels several hundred thousand times below most national safety limits (including Canada's).

The BioInitiative scientists believe that there may be NO safe lower exposure limits! Research has found that proximity to power lines (extremely low frequency EMF) causes childhood cancers, such as leukemia. High frequency EMF exposures, such as occur with frequent use of cell phones, cause cancer (e.g., acoustic neuroma) in children and adults. Further, there is evidence that exposure is associated with neurodegenerative diseases such as Amyotrophic Lateral Sclerosis (ALS) and Alzheimer's Disease. Both low and high frequency EMF damage DNA, provoke cells to make heat shock proteins (something they do when stressed), and negatively impact the immune system. The reports raise some very interesting and provocative concerns that should not be ignored.

SYMPTOMS OF ELECTRO HYPERSENSITIVITY					
Neurological		**Cardiac**	**Respiratory**	**Dermatological**	**Ophthalmologic**
headaches	depression	palpitations	sinusitis	skin rash	deteriorating vision
difficulty concentrating	anxiety	pain or pressure in the chest	asthma	facial flushing	pain or burning in the eyes
muscle and joint pain	confusion and spatial disorientation	low or high blood pressure	bronchitis	itching	pressure in/behind the eyes
memory loss	fatigue	shortness of breath	pneumonia	burning	floaters
dizziness	weakness	arrhythmias			cataracts
nausea	tremors	slow or fast heart rate		swelling of face and neck	
irritability	muscle spasms				
numbness	leg/foot pain				
tingling	"Flu-like" symptoms				
hyperactivity	fever				
altered reflexes	insomnia				
OTHER					
digestive problems	abdominal pain	testicular/ovarian pain/swelling	enlarged thyroid	great thirst	dehydration
nosebleeds	internal bleeding	hair loss	pain in the teeth	deteriorating fillings	Light sensitivity
swollen lymph nodes	loss of appetite	hypoxia	allergies	frequent urination and incontinence	night sweats
immune abnormalities	redistribution of metals within the body	ringing in the ears (tinnitus or similar chronic ear-noise)	impaired sense of smell	altered sugar metabolism	dryness of lips, tongue, mouth, eyes
Severe reactions can include seizures, paralysis, psychosis, and stroke					

Symptoms of Electro Hypersensivity
This chart is from the WEEP Initiative EHS Survival Guide and is used with permission of the author, Sue Parsons.

Symptoms of EHS

The list of symptoms above is taken from the Canadian Initiative to Stop Wireless, Electric, and Electromagnetic Pollution (WEEP) *EHS Survival Guide* (Parsons, 2007). You can see that the symptoms are extremely diverse. Diagnosis depends upon close observation of whether symptoms worsen when you are in proximity to EMF and lessen when you move farther away. The intensity of electromagnetic fields decreases by the square of the distance from the source.

The primary "treatment" of EHS is to avoid exposure. The Survival Guide has good information in that regard. I don't recommend the parts of the report on other treatment strategies, as there is currently no evidence to support that any of these suggestions work. They reflect the opinion and experience of the author and are certainly deserving of further study. While some of the recommendations may be helpful, there is, as of yet, no research to substantiate the benefits of any medical or nutritional treatments for EHS.

How to Identify and Avoid Electromagnetic Risks

EMF emanates in all directions from every source; it goes through walls, combines with other sources, etc. There are NO rules of thumb on what is safe without measuring a specific location at various times of the day and night. This is because the amount of electromagnetic flow on wired and wireless networks is constantly changing. Also, each EMF wave interacts with each other when they meet, and the waves can cancel each other out, be additive, or create new frequencies. In other words, one cannot say that living a certain distance from a high voltage power line will be safe without both measurement and careful observation by the persons who may be affected.

I've discussed some of the useful tools for measuring EMF at the end of Session 5 (in the section, Preparing for Session 6), but here is a summary. An Amp/Voltmeter can be used to measure *Body Voltage* (the amount of EMF actually entering your body). The safe level of Body Voltage is less than 100mV. There is also a *TriField meter,* which measures both electrical and magnetic fields. On this analogue meter, the "unsafe range" is indicated by a red line. Safe measurements are those that don't go into the "red." Specialized radiofrequency detectors detect wireless and radio frequencies. The safe limit is thought to be below 1 microWatt/m2. This is the lowest measurable reading on the meter I use in the office. These are rough tools. If you have significant symptoms, you will need to hire an electrician or building biologist with training in the field and high-end equipment.

Common Sources of EMF

- Electrical wiring: Even when an appliance is turned off, electricity still runs through the wires.
- Fluorescent and LED light bulbs and light dimmers are especially problematic because of fluctuating fields. If you hold a TriField meter up to a compact fluorescent light bulb, you can see the needle move back and forth at the frequency of the bulb.
- All electrical appliances, including battery-operated ones like your bedside alarm clock.
- All wireless transmitters and receivers, such as cordless phones, wireless mice and keyboards, cell phones, and in-home Wi-Fi, should be turned off when not in use. Very sensitive individuals will need to avoid them altogether.
- All the electrical wiring and instrumentation in vehicles, as well as the magnetic field from the motor. This magnetic field is much higher in hybrid vehicles.
- Medical imaging equipment such as X-rays, CT, and MRI scans.

Ways of Lowering EMF Exposure

- Don't use wireless devices such as hands-free, cell and smartphones, or limit their use.
- Turn off all electronics not in use.
- Identify hot spots in your house, and when possible, turn off the electricity to those areas at the electrical panel.
- Don't keep any electrical devices in your bedroom. EMF interferes with melatonin production and with restorative sleep.
- Ensure that you sit at a safe distance from computers, TVs, etc. This can only be established by measuring the EMF.
- Replace fluorescent and LED light bulbs with incandescent or halogen bulbs.
- Don't move to a house/apartment in proximity to cell towers or high-voltage power lines. Again, one must measure to determine what a safe distance is.
- If you can, don't allow smart meters to be installed in your house. They emit very low power fields, but for highly sensitive individuals, they may have an impact. More study is certainly needed before they are mandated for installation in every home in Canada, as is currently occurring.

Avoiding EMF is becoming increasingly difficult. The City of Calgary has endorsed a city-wide installation of Wi-Fi transmitters on lamp posts and the replacement of all utility meters with smart meters. Similar transitions are in progress across Canada. In response to what they see, organizations are forming to inform and fight a looming public health disaster. One such group is Citizens for Safe Technology, a BC based group. Their website is www.citizensforsafetechnology.com. Another source of information is Dr. Magda Havas's (an Associate Professor of Environmental & Resource Studies at Trent University) website at http://www.magdahavas.com/.

In Feb. 2012, the Health and Safety Committee of the Ontario English Catholic Teachers' Association (OECTA) issued a position paper outlining the health concerns associated with Wi-Fi in schools, which many have interpreted as calling for a moratorium on their use. Responses to their paper have been mixed, with many supporting the idea of a ban while others, government and press alike, expressing the view that this is fearmongering and misinformation. Like much in science, there is still much to be discovered.

Preparing for Session 7

Before reading the next session on pain, it is strongly recommended that you spend 2 weeks focusing your attention on all the types of pain that you have. Your focus should be on noticing what makes each pain worse or better.

You will need the following:

- Sleep Chart or Activity and Symptoms Chart.

Joan has already learned some things about her pain. The charts completed in Sessions 1 and 3 reveal that her daily pain level ranges from 3 - 8/10. Her pain is generally higher when her energy is lower (Sleep Chart Session 1). And her pain also seems to be higher when she is stressed (Sleep Chart Session 3). However, Joan has several types of pain, and these charts don't differentiate between them. The objective in the next 2 weeks is to identify each type of pain and the triggering activities for each.

To notice the impact of certain activities on each pain type, Joan used the Activity and Symptoms Chart, and she concentrated on pain. She used the same chart in preparation for this session (6), but in that case, she used the chart to observe time-related symptoms of environmental exposures.

Activity and Symptoms Chart

Name: Joan Smith Date Feb 13/12 to Feb 26/12

Date & Time	Activity	Symptom
Feb 13/12	rested	stiff + sore all over.
Daily	walk dog	stiff to start, then feel better, then ↑ pain as walk continues.
Feb 14	dinner out	bowel cramps + diarrhea for several hours.
Feb 17	upsetting call from friend → worry → bad sleep	↑ muscle tension + pain × 3 days.
Feb 20	sitting for > 1 hr doing paperwork	↑ pain in mid-upper back
Feb 22	massage	↓ pain × 2 days
Feb 24	housework incl. vacuuming	↑ sore + stiff all over muscle fatigue
Feb 25	epsom salt bath	warm + relaxed
Feb 26	attended church (perfume exposure)	headache + fatigue

Session 6 References

Genuis, S. J., Beesoon, S., Birkholz, D., & Lobo, R. A. (2012). Human excretion of bisphenol A: blood, urine, and sweat (BUS) study. *J Environ. Public Health, 2012,* 185731. doi:https://onlinelibrary.wiley.com/doi/10.1155/2012/185731

Genuis, S. J., Beesoon, S., Lobo, R. A., & Birkholz, D. (2012). Human Elimination of Phthalate Compounds: Blood, Urine, and Sweat (BUS) Study. *The Scientific World Journal, 2012,* 10. doi:https://onlinelibrary.wiley.com/doi/10.1100/2012/615068

Genuis, S. J., Birkholz, D., Rodushkin, I., & Beesoon, S. (2011). Blood, urine, and sweat (BUS) study: monitoring and elimination of bioaccumulated toxic elements. *Arch. Environ. Contam Toxicol, 61*(2), 344–357. doi:https://www.researchgate.net/publication/47701626_Blood_Urine_and_Sweat_BUS_Study_Monitoring_and_Elimination_of_Bioaccumulated_Toxic_Elements

Hamilton, M. J. (2018). Nonclonal Mast Cell Activation Syndrome: A Growing Body of Evidence. *Immunology & Allergy Clinics of North America, 38*(3), 469–481. doi:https://dx.doi.org/10.1016/j.iac.2018.04.002

Hussain, J., & Cohen, M. (2018). Clinical Effects of Regular Dry Sauna Bathing: A Systematic Review. *Evidence-Based Complementary and Alternative Medicine, 2018,* 30. doi:https://www.researchgate.net/publication/322509545_Clinical_Effects_of_Regular_Dry_Sauna_Bathing_A_Systematic_Review

Marshall, L., Bested, A., J., M., Kerr, K., & Bray, R. (2011). *Environmental Sensitivities-Multiple Chemical Sensitivities Status Report.* Retrieved from Toronto, Canada: http://www.womenshealthmatters.ca/assets/legacy/wch/pdfs/ESMCSStatusReportJune22011.pdf

Patrick, R. P., & Johnson, T. L. (2021). Sauna use as a lifestyle practice to extend healthspan. *Experimental Gerontology, 154,* 111509. doi:https://doi.org/10.1016/j.exger.2021.111509

Sears, M. E. (2007). *The Medical Perspective on Environmental Sensitivities.* Retrieved from Ottawa, Canada: https://publications.gc.ca/site/eng/9.691154/publication.html

Valent, P., Akin, C., Bonadonna, P., Hartmann, K., Brockow, K., Niedoszytko, M., . . . Metcalfe, D. D. (2019). Proposed Diagnostic Algorithm for Patients with Suspected Mast Cell Activation Syndrome. *The Journal of Allergy & Clinical Immunology in Practice, 7*(4), 1125–1133.e1121. doi:https://dx.doi.org/10.1016/j.jaip.2019.01.006

Wilkie, C., & Baker, D. (2008). *Accommodation for Environmental Sensitivities: Legal Perspective.* Retrieved from Ottawa, Canada: https://publications.gc.ca/site/eng/332178/publication.html

Session 7

Pain Management

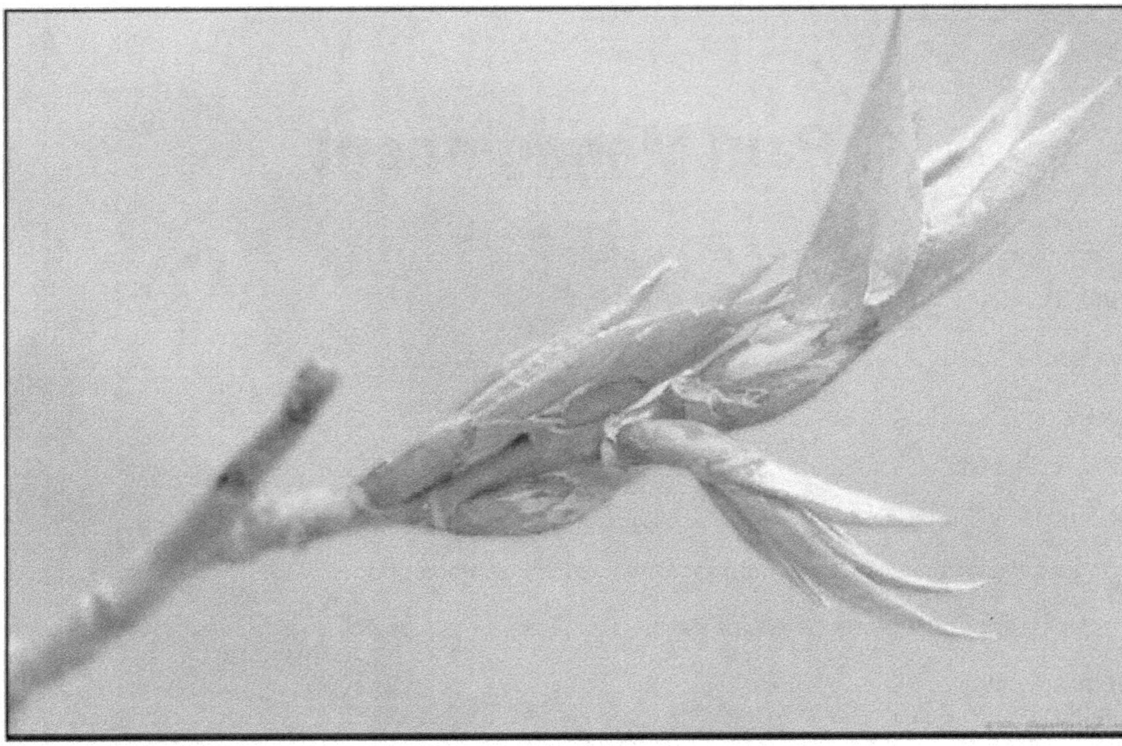

Life Line

Life Line

I was walking through the woods around Wedge Pond when I saw this twig. It seemed to be filling with life after a hard winter. I felt like it was like **my** life line. I have been ill for a while and am becoming more active and feeling better. The vestigial branch of the twig represents my illness; dark, unfocused, digressing from the right path. The right branch is the one filling with new growth, joy, color and purpose...like a new lease on life. You will notice the growth is in several directions, green growing from a red (painful) base, branching out into the sunlight. You will also notice that the ends of the new leaves are unfocused...I'm not sure where I'm heading, but it all looks good!

Session 7

Pain Management

Objectives

- To increase knowledge about normal and pathological pain in people with ME/CFS, FM and MCS.
- To improve self-management of pain.
- To learn about interventions (including medication) to maximize quality of life despite chronic pain.

Introduction

Pain is the primary symptom in fibromyalgia. It is also common in myalgic encephalomyelitis /chronic fatigue syndrome and can occur in multiple chemical sensitivity or in people who do not meet the full criteria for MCS, as part of a chemical sensitivity reaction. In this session, I will be referring primarily to the muscle pain and stiffness experienced in fibromyalgia. However, most patients with ME/CFS, FM and MCS also experience other types of pain such as migraine headaches, pain from irritable bowel syndrome, pelvic pain, or arthritis pain. These other types of pain are also important to address, but are not dealt with in this session.

The clinical suggestions in this session are based on pain literature and my clinical experience. This session, in common with the other sessions, is not an exhaustive list of all helpful strategies. Also, in common with the other sessions, many of these strategies help in certain individuals, but no one strategy will help everyone.

Here are some philosophical points that guide my thinking about pain:

1. The primary objective in the management of chronic pain is to increase daily functioning. In most cases, only partial improvement in pain levels is possible. However, increasing function and quality of life is virtually always possible.

2. Getting better requires an active approach on your part. There are no drugs or interventions that will decrease or eliminate your pain without your active participation. Active participation means examining your lifestyle, attitudes, and activities and being willing to make changes where necessary. This often

includes charting to identify your pain patterns, identifying your pain window (similar in concept to the energy envelope) and then making changes to your life to prevent pain spikes.

3. Changes are easier to make when one understands that, in most cases, chronic pain is due to changes in the neurological pain pathways and not damage to the tissues themselves. The book *Explain Pain* is an excellent pictorial guide to the physiology of chronic pain (Butler et al., 2003). If you are afraid to make changes for fear of making your pain worse, I strongly recommend this book and the resources on the Neuro-orthopaedic Institute website at http://www.noigroup.com/en/Home. Both are good introductions to making neuroplasticity (the brain's ability to change) work for you.

4. Recovery from disability caused by chronic pain requires an open mind. You may need to try several approaches until you find one that works. If you give up after a few strategies have failed to work, you are selling yourself short.

Pain Physiology

This section provides a very basic introduction to the processes and functions involved in pain, including a few definitions commonly used in any discussion about pain.

- **Hyperalgesia or pain hypersensitivity:** Refers to increased pain intensity and/or prolonged pain duration evoked by stimuli that are normally painful.
- **Allodynia:** Refers to pain elicited by normally non-painful stimuli such as light touch.
- **Neuropathic or nerve pain:** This is pain that is caused by the nerves themselves as opposed to other tissues, bone, organs, etc. Neuropathic pain is thought to reflect either damage to the nerves, as in the case of diabetes, or changes in nerve transmission, as is thought to be the case in fibromyalgia. Increasingly, fibromyalgia is classified as a type of neuropathic pain.

Neuroplasticity

When I went to medical school, we were taught that the brain couldn't change. If it was injured, for example, by a stroke, little recovery was possible. However, this is simply not true. We now have enormous evidence to support that the brain is constantly adapting to the signals it receives from the environment and the body. If signals change, the brain starts remodelling almost immediately, and measurable changes can be found within 5 days. This ability to change is called *neuroplasticity*. Neuroplasticity can cause problems, such as chronic pain, but it also gives hope of solutions to problems that were, until recently, thought to be unsolvable.

Acute pain can cause changes in neurons that increase the risk of developing chronic pain. For example, poor pain management after injury or surgery increases the chances of developing chronic pain. The chronic pain does not mean that the original injury hasn't healed. Rather, most chronic pain is the result of changes to the pain pathways and even changes to the anatomy of the nerves running between the area of initial injury and the pain-processing centers in the brain. It is, in some cases, an "illusion" of pain—perceived as real enough but nevertheless, an "illusion."

Novel approaches to the treatment of chronic pain involve using neuroplasticity for benefit. The book, *The Brain that Changes Itself,* by Toronto psychiatrist Dr. Norman Doidge, explains some of the amazing advances being made to utilize the brain's plasticity to heal from any number of health problems, including chronic pain (Doidge, 2007). Doidge introduces an approach to phantom limb pain that involves tricking the body into believing the limb (no longer present) is moving and receiving impulses. You can view a program about Dr. Doidge's book on *The Nature of Things* with Dr. David Suzuki at the CBC website link https://www.youtube.com/watch?v=VIdWFuuZaxw

Dr. V.S. Ramachandran is the scientist who developed the novel approach to phantom limb pain described in Dr. Doidge's book. He explains that chronic pain is actually an illusion—the body is misinterpreting the signals it is receiving. His approach to phantom limb pain and other chronic pain is an attempt to trick the body back into a non-pain interpretation by generating new neural pathways that do not involve pain.

For more on the application of Dr. Ramachandran's work, there is an interesting YouTube video by a therapist using mirrors to trick the brain into developing non-pain pathways at http://www.youtube.com/watch?v=jp8QZ6L59J4. This is very exciting work that could revolutionize the management of chronic pain.

Since writing the previous section on neuroplasticity, the field of using neuroplasticity as a tool for healing has exploded. Rather than editing this chapter, which remains accurate and useful, I have added a bonus chapter introducing some of the new approaches.

Normal Pain Processing

Painful stimuli such as pressure, temperature, or inflammation are sensed by sensory nerves at the site of the injury. Pain signals travel along the peripheral nerves (mostly A delta and C fibres) to the spinal cord, where they connect with nerves that travel to the brain. Nerve signals can be augmented or inhibited (made more or less strong) at every synapse (connection) along the way.

Using brain imaging techniques such as Positron Emission Tomography (PET) and Functional Magnetic Resonance Imaging (fMRI), the normal pain pathways in the brain have been identified. Pain processing is multifaceted and involves many parts of the brain. A division can be found between the areas processing sensory and discriminative aspects of pain (i.e., where the pain is and what type of pain is felt) and the emotional aspects of pain. Both the sensory/discriminative and the emotional facets influence pain perception. If healthy, the brain and spinal cord continually send signals from the brain down to the extremities to block or decrease excessive pain signals. This is called descending inhibition.

Neurotransmitters and Neural Pathways Involved in Pain Perception

Brain cells (neurons) communicate by exchanging signals (either electrical or chemical) across synapses (the gaps where the neurons meet). The signals can be either excitatory (up-regulating) or inhibitory (down-regulating). The signals are transmitted from one neuron by a neurotransmitter and are received by the receptor of a nearby neuron. The transmitters and receptors are specific (i.e., endorphins bind to opioid receptors, not to serotonin receptors).

The study of neurotransmitters has been useful in developing many pain medications. In other cases, many drugs were found by accident to be helpful for chronic pain, and it was only later that the connection to a particular neurotransmitter was understood. Pain drugs are discussed later in this session.

- Serotonin, dopamine, and noradrenaline are all involved with pain transmission and perception. Altered levels of these transmitters are thought to be associated with chronic pain conditions such as FM. Treatments such as older tricyclic antidepressants (e.g., amitriptyline) increase neurotransmitter levels and decrease pain perception. Some serotonin (5-HT) receptors increase pain (5-HT3), whereas some decrease pain perception (5-HT1A). While very useful for other purposes (e.g., sleep, depression), I have not found the serotonin drugs, such as the selective serotonin antidepressants (SSRIs), useful as pain medicine.
- N-Methyl-D-aspartate (NMDA) receptors are thought to be strongly connected with pain in general and the pain response in people with FM in particular. Ketamine, a drug usually used during anaesthesia, is an NMDA receptor blocker. When used intramuscularly, ketamine has been shown to dramatically reduce pain in patients with FM (Graven-Nielsen et al., 2000). Ketamine is not available in oral form, and injectable forms are dangerous. But new dermal preparations are being used with success.
- Gamma-aminobutyric acid (GABA), the neurotransmitter stimulated by diazepam (Valium®), can increase or decrease pain perception depending upon the concentration and circumstances. Newer pain medications such as gabapentin (Neurontin®) and pregabalin (Lyrica®) are GABA analogues. They act by binding to voltage-gated calcium receptors, thereby decreasing excitatory neurotransmitter (e.g., NMDA) release.
- The body makes marijuana like neurotransmitters which act on the CB1 and CB2 receptors in the brain. Δ9-tetrahydrocannabinol (THC), the active component in marijuana, acts at the endogenous cannabinoid receptors and has effects on thinking and pain.

Joan's Activity and Symptoms Chart for Pain

For this next section, you will need to refer to both Joan's and your Activity and Symptoms Charts regarding pain (Session 6). You may also want to review Joan's Sleep Charts in Sessions 1 and 3, as they rate her pain at that time.

Looking at Joan's Sleep Charts (Session 1 and Session 3), we can see that her daily pain level ranges from 3 - 8/10. We can also see that her pain seems to be higher when her energy is lower (Sleep Chart Session 1) and when she is stressed (Sleep Chart Session 3). However, Joan has several types of pain, and these charts don't differentiate between them. This is clearer on her Activity and Symptoms Chart (which she completed in Session 6).

In her most recent charting, Joan identifies four distinct types of pain:

- Ankle pain: It's described as throbbing, constant, and worse with standing or walking. Joan makes a note to talk to her family physician at the next appointment to see if there is any treatment for her ankle pain, even though it is an injury from several years previous.
- Headache pain: By the end of this charting period, Joan realizes that she could take some steps to lessen her headache pain by decreasing her exposure to fragrances. She is considering wearing a mask or convincing her boss and the minister at church to agree to a "no scent" policy.
- Bowel pain: This severe cramping pain is not frequent and seems related to eating certain foods or to being exposed to chemicals. Joan still isn't certain what the triggers are.
- Muscle pain: Joan always has some background dull, aching, tiring muscle pain. So far, she has identified that this pain is worse when she is stressed and/or doesn't get a good sleep. She refers to this as FM pain.

You can see that after several weeks of charting, Joan is starting to notice patterns and is attempting interventions. Some of them are working. This increases her sense of empowerment and hope. As Joan works through this manual, she discovers that her ankle pain is a *peripheral pain generator* and that if she could lessen this pain, it may help with her FM pain.

Look at your own charts, including your Sleep charts from Sessions 1 and 3. What kinds of pain do you have? Are there any patterns that you notice or triggers that you can identify? Read on to get more ideas as to what you might be able to do.

Pain in Fibromyalgia

What Does FM Pain Feel Like?

Not all pain feels the same. The most common descriptors of FM pain are that it is most intense in large muscles such as the thighs and upper back. FM pain typically worsens with repetitive activity and is relieved by rest. People use adjectives such as "aching," "tiring," or "heavy" to describe FM pain. Arthritis pain is often described as "deep," "sharp," or "bone" pain. Non-FM neuropathic pain is most often described as "burning," "tingling," or "shooting." Infectious pain is described as "tender" or "throbbing."

Where Does FM Pain Come From?

Although not conclusively proven, research suggests that even though it feels as if it is coming from the muscles, much of the pain in ME/CFS, FM and MCS is caused by the spinal cord and brain through a process referred to as *central sensitization* (Yunus, 2007). When people say that FM is all in the head, they may be correct, but not for the reasons they thought.

With central sensitization, the *pain volume* is turned up in the brain and spinal cord. It is thought that this same mechanism may explain the pain in ME/CFS, Irritable Bowel Syndrome (IBS), migraine headaches, interstitial cystitis, and other conditions. This central pain explanation is good news since it may be amenable to some of the neuroplasticity techniques being introduced.

Other authors, such as Dr. Roland Staud, believe that both central and peripheral mechanisms influence pain perception in FM (Staud, 2010). His view is supported by a study that showed that FM pain disappeared entirely with an injection of painkillers into the fluid around the spinal cord. This suggests that some of the pain is produced outside the brain.

Other causes of pain, such as trauma or disease (e.g., arthritis or an injury), probably don't cause FM but may precipitate and perpetuate any chronic pain problem. These are called *Peripheral Pain Generators* and need to be optimally treated to improve pain in people with FM. In summary, both central and peripheral mechanisms are thought to influence pain perception in FM. Either way, chronic pain should be amenable to strategies that utilize neuroplasticity.

FM Pain Is Real and Measurable

In a recent review of pain imaging in FM, Dr. Dane Cook and colleagues concluded that the evidence for abnormal pain processing in FM is strong. Some of the specific studies are mentioned in the following section. The types of abnormal pain processing fall into the following categories (Cook et al., 2007):

- Dysregulation of descending inhibition from the brain (go back to the discussion about normal pain processing at the beginning of this session, if this doesn't mean anything to you). In FM, these inhibitory signals from the brain are decreased.
- Augmented "wind-up" and delayed after-sensations to repetitive stimuli: In healthy people, after a pain stimulus, the central nervous system (brain and spinal cord) inhibits further signals. This is why healthy people can distract themselves from one pain by self-inflicting another (e.g., squeezing or biting one's hand when getting an injection). In FM, the opposite happens. Each pain stimulus sensitizes the system so that the pain signals ramp up or "wind up." In FM, successive signals are increasingly painful. Also, pain lasts longer in people with FM when compared to healthy controls.
- Absence of exercise-induced analgesic effect: In healthy individuals, exercise decreases pain perception. The endorphins that are produced during exercise exert an endogenous painkiller effect. This explains why athletes can continue to compete despite severe injuries. In FM, response to pain increases rather than decreases after exercise. This abnormal response is also found in ME/CFS.

Key Imaging Studies in FM

Studies show decreased brain blood flow to specific parts of the brain in subjects with FM compared with healthy controls. These brain areas include most of the areas known to be involved in pain processing, providing strong evidence that FM has a biological underpinning.

In response to painful stimuli such as thumb pressure, heat or cold, people with FM show increased brain reactivity (Gracely et al., 2002). This objectively measured response corresponds with subjective reports of increased pain in patients with FM when compared to healthy controls. In addition, some areas of the brain, such as the thalamus and periaqueductal gray matter, which are activated in healthy people exposed to pain, fail to activate in people with FM. This is thought to explain the decrease in descending inhibition found in FM.

It has been shown that pain catastrophizing (panicking about one's pain) is related to increased activity in both sensory and affective processing areas of the brain (Nijs et al., 2008). In other words, fear makes pain feel worse. Similarly, depression increases sensitivity to the affective component of pain as viewed on brain imaging (Bushnell et al., 2002; Giesecke et al., 2005).

There are only a few treatment studies using imaging to evaluate the impact of treatment on pain. In one study, patients with FM were treated with 25 mg amitriptyline for 3 months. Their self-reported pain decreased, and blood flow to the thalamus increased compared with the pre-treatment assessment (Adiguzel et al., 2004). A small study using electroshock treatment had similar results.

Lastly, using a new technology, Voxel Based Morphometry (MR-VBM), the brains of patients with FM and other chronic pain disorders have been found to be smaller in some areas than the brains of healthy controls (May, 2008). The brain changes correlate with both pain and fatigue symptoms (Lutz et al., 2008). Similar loss of brain volume is found in other chronic pain conditions and in ME/CFS. It may reflect a lack of use of those parts of the brain. Plasticity means that we truly "use it or lose it" when it comes to the brain. In ME/CFS, it has been shown that with therapy, the brain volume can recover, suggesting that the loss of volume is not due to neuronal death but rather neuroplasticity at work (de Lange et al., 2008).

Why Aren't These Objective Tests Available to Patients?

I am frequently asked why, if there are so many tools to measure abnormalities in pain perception objectively, patients don't have access to these tests. Objective measurements would make the lives of most FM patients much easier as they would be more likely to be believed by others, including their physicians.

Here is the answer to this question. In FM research, groups of patients are compared with groups of healthy people of similar age and fitness levels. The studies consistently show differences between groups of individuals, but in a given individual, test results are not reliable.

The diagram below shows considerable overlap in the test results of healthy people and ill individuals. In other words, some patients fit the healthy profile, and some healthy people fit the pain/FM profile. This means that if such a test were used widely in clinical practice, there would be both false positive and false negative results. Until a test is 99% or more accurate in discriminating between people who are healthy and people who are ill, it isn't ready for clinical use and cannot be considered a reliable marker for a condition. Sometimes it is possible to improve the odds by combining several tests; however, this adds to the cost. So far, all the imaging tests used in FM research are quite expensive and time-consuming, making them poor candidates to be used in combination with an illness as common as FM.

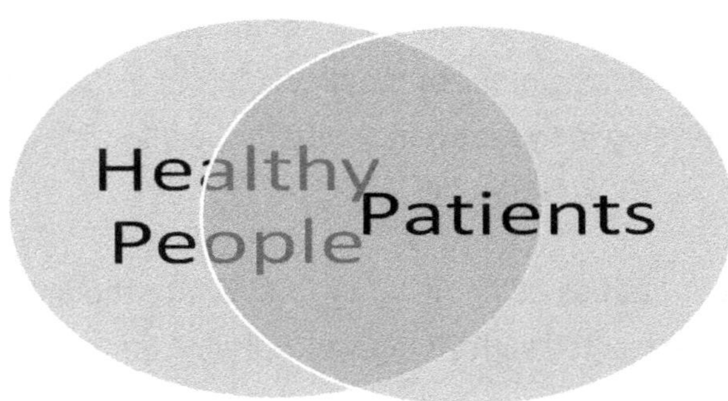

Test results overlap between healthy people and patients. Therefore, if a test result came back in the darkened overlapping zone, one would not be able to determine from the result whether someone has the disorder in question (e.g., chronic pain).

Is the Pain in FM Similar to That in Other Chronic Pain Conditions?

Imaging studies show similarities between function in the brains of patients with FM and Irritable Bowel Syndrome (IBS), whereas patients with Rheumatoid Arthritis show a different profile. In a study comparing chronic lower back pain and FM, subjects were exposed to sub-painful pressure stimuli—a level of stimulation that healthy people do not find painful.

Both of these chronic pain groups showed brain activation in the pain regions of the brain when exposed to low-level stimulation, suggesting some common physiology at play between different types of chronic pain. FM patients show a stronger affective (mood) response to pain than other chronic pain groups. This leads some to suggest that there is a stronger connection between FM and mood disorders than with other chronic pain conditions. The connection between mood and ME/CFS and FM will be discussed further in Session 8.

Pain Management

There are very few studies that report the use of objective measures before and after treatment. Most studies of chronic pain, including drug studies, compare patients' subjective perceptions of pain, function, and other measures before and after the treatment in question. However, there are some studies that have used objective scans as a way to measure treatment. I've already mentioned one of these studies in the key imaging section. This study shows that successful treatment of chronic pain is associated with improvement of Single-Photon Emission Computed Tomography (SPECT) scan abnormalities (Adiguzel et al., 2004).

This suggests that the brain changes in FM are not necessarily permanent. A recent study showed that patients with FM can learn to modulate their pain pathways using fMRI as a tool. EEG biofeedback is increasingly available as a tool for several conditions, including FM. My impression of this treatment is mixed, with some people benefiting and others getting inexplicably worse.

Lifestyle Interventions: Finding a Balance

Pain is a symptom very much affected by lifestyle, attitude, mood, and stress levels. Daily charting will assist you in identifying the factors that are associated with increases or decreases in your pain. These factors may not be apparent without careful observation. For example, in many patients, food or chemical exposures increase pain, especially headache pain.

Many of the same strategies that you have already been using to economize your energy will also help you manage pain. It's all about balance. Remember that your goal is long-term improvement—you must be strategic to reach this. Here are some tips on pacing your activity levels to minimize pain spikes:

- Avoiding activity for fear of increasing pain leads to decreased fitness, increased stiffness, and reduced pain thresholds. In other words, too much avoidance for fear of having more pain leads to more pain. Whoops! In the diagram below, avoidance is called the "wait until" approach.
- On the other hand, an approach of pushing through the pain no matter what leads to frequent pain spikes, which can take too long to resolve. Over the long term, this also leads to increased pain. In my practice, this is the hardest lesson for patients to learn. Patients repeatedly overdo their activity level and are then surprised that their pain increases...every time. In the diagram below, this approach is referred to as "do it no matter what."
- Most chronic pain specialists recommend a stepwise progression of activity using body symptoms as a biofeedback measure. If pacing optimally for your health levels, overall pain levels will decrease over time. If your pain is increasing, you may consider changing your strategy.

The diagram below illustrates the three behavioral patterns for dealing with pain just summarized. You will see that the pacing approach, though the activity level starts lower, ends with a much higher capability than either of the other two approaches.

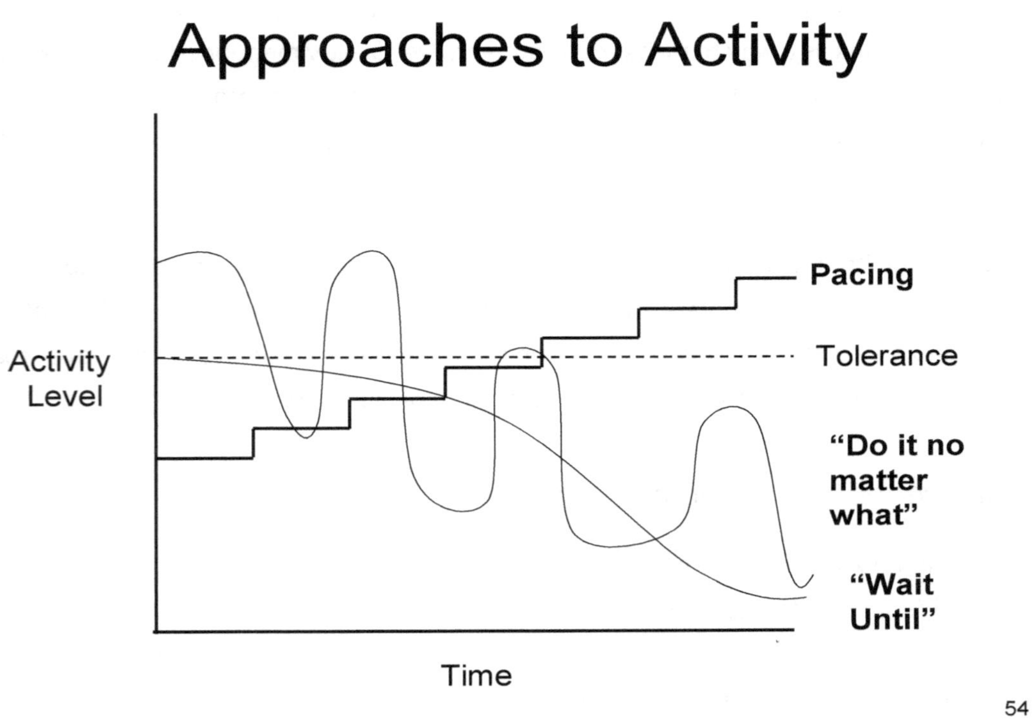

This figure was developed by staff at the Calgary Chronic Pain Centre and is used with permission.

- As with finding your energy envelope in Session 3, the starting point for a pacing program is generally less than what you are currently doing.
- Start with an activity level and pacing strategy that doesn't increase your baseline pain in any day by more than 2/10 on a 10-point scale. If your pain increases more than 2/10, the cost will likely outweigh the benefits.
- As with energy pacing, at first, your limitations may feel very depressing. You will want to be doing more. But if your goal is long-term sustainable improvement, you may be willing to sacrifice some of the immediate gratification of getting tasks done faster or doing things independently.
- With FM pain, it is important to avoid excessive repetition of a single movement. For example, if swimming, one should rotate the strokes to avoid tiring one muscle group excessively.
- You may find that paying attention to the ergonomics of an activity is helpful. In other words, there may be one aspect of an activity that increases pain. If you are able to identify this by breaking the activity down into parts, you might be able to think of a way to do the offending part differently.
- You may find that the use of a heart rate monitor and the pacing strategies you have been using to maintain your energy levels will also help with pain management. If so, an HR monitor can be a useful tool to remind you when you are on a path of overactivity.

It may be necessary to obtain expert advice when trying to sort out what types of activities to do and how many of them to do. Most physiotherapists and kinesiologists have the skills needed to help you set up an individual exercise program. In choosing a physiotherapist or kinesiologist, it is recommended that you ensure that they are knowledgeable about your condition (ME/CFS, FM and/or MCS) or that they are willing to learn.

Behavioral Interventions

Any psychological intervention that increases the ability to cope with loss, stress, and uncertainty has the potential to benefit people with chronic pain or, for that matter, with any chronic condition. Empowerment or feeling in charge of one's own health makes a big difference. Increasing your sense of empowerment is the primary objective of this manual. By identifying things that make you feel better and doing more of them to improve health and functioning, you will begin to feel more empowered and hopeful that you can have a better life.

1. Managing anxiety and fear is an important part of pain management. Anxiety and fear are the opposite of empowerment. They are the belief that one's fate rests with external factors and that nothing except hiding and avoiding will lead to improvement. Anxiety and fear increase perceived pain severity. Anxiety and fear can only be remedied by facing them head-on. *Feel the Fear and Do it Anyway* by Dr. Susan Jeffers is a good guide for those who are freaking out at this last statement (Jeffers, 2007).

Facing fears and working through them involves purposely engaging in the feared behavior or situation to see what happens. This requires real-life exposure to the feared event while at the same time having practiced the skills needed to ride out the wave of fear that will be triggered. It will pass. Once the wave of fear has passed, one realizes that the feared situation can be tolerated. With practice, it will become easier and easier until it ceases to be feared at all. Another book I recommend is the *Anxiety and Phobia Workbook* by Dr. Edmund Bourne (Bourne, 2001). You'll also see this book recommended in Session 8. As well, many of the coping strategies discussed in Session 4 are of value as part of your pain management toolkit.

2. Mindfulness meditation, such as the Mindfulness-Based Stress Reduction (MBSR) discussed in Session 4, has been shown to improve depression in people with FM, but the effects of meditation on pain are less clear. Mindfulness meditation involves concentrated focus on breathing. Over time, practitioners of meditation are able to affect their autonomic responses. Increased heart rate and breathing rate associated with anxiety, anger, and frustration all increase pain.

Interventions such as timed breathing and meditation, which decrease adrenaline response, will moderate pain. These skills must be practised regularly to be mastered. They will not work the first time you try them. Consistent practice based on the instruction of a book, video, or trained instructor will lead to improved skill. If you are interested in this approach, I would recommend the Mindfulness-Based Stress Reduction (MBSR) information at the University of Massachusetts Medical School website at https://www.ummhealth.org/services-treatments/center-mindfulness/mindfulness-programs/mbsr.

3. Self-hypnosis is a variant of the meditation method, which is commonly used for pain management. Self-hypnosis involves focus on a script or visualization, which contains the suggestion of the ability to cope with pain, reframed meaning of pain, and evaporation of pain, etc. A study has shown that SPECT scans can change when a subject undergoes hypnotically induced analgesia. This suggests that hypnosis can actually change pain perception at a central and biological level.

All these interventions require willingness and motivation to practice, and belief that they may work, in other words, an active approach. None of these interventions will cure the pain, but they can decrease the sensation of pain and secondary augmentation caused by anxiety. Maybe these approaches help in part through neuroplasticity, forming new neural pathways that don't involve pain but rather relaxation.

Treating Peripheral Pain Generators

People with ME/CFS, FM and MCS may have injuries or diseases that cause pain apart from the fatiguing disorder. Examples include recent surgery, fracture or other injury, burn, arthritis, or acute or chronic infection. These peripheral pain generators are not usually the cause of FM pain (though they may be the trigger), but unless treated, they can perpetuate FM pain. In Joan's case, her ankle injury is a chronic peripheral pain generator.

Physical Therapies

- Some patients with FM pain find that heat gives temporary relief. Heating pads can be used as long as they are not left on for long periods of time or are hot enough to cause burns or electrical fires. Home hot tubs are used by some patients, as well as exercise in warm water pools. This last method, called *balneotherapy,* has been formally assessed and found to be helpful for pain, but not mood, in a small European study.
- Home Transcutaneous Electric Nerve Stimulation (TENS) machines are also helpful for some patients. This has not been formally studied and is anecdotal only. The rapidly alternating electrical current causes muscles to feel numb and relaxed. This strategy may help temporarily decrease pain in tense, painful muscles.
- Physiotherapy, chiropractic, massage therapy, acupuncture, intramuscular stimulation, yoga, and bioenergetic therapies can all be helpful for people with pain due to ME/CFS, FM and MCS. However, without active management (something you do yourself), the relief will be temporary.
- Physical therapies are effective for many peripheral pain syndromes (e.g., arthritis, tendonitis, injury). Physical therapies tend to retain their benefits much more in people who are also practising self-management skills.
- Restorative, active treatment, such as core stabilization exercises, can increase the strength of the core muscles and decrease the demand on the peripheral muscles, which are perceived as painful in FM. Pilates is one such approach. Patients should start slowly, ideally with an instructor with some knowledge of FM, to avoid overdoing it.
- As noted in relation to physiotherapists and kinesiologists, all physical therapies must be adapted to fit the pain thresholds and energy levels of patients with ME/CFS, FM and MCS to have any chance of success. If any professional encourages you to push through the pain, you might need to find someone else to work with.

Pain Medications

The goal of using pain medication may include any or all of the following:

- To increase quality of life.
- To increase functional capacity.
- To improve sleep.
- To prevent the development of secondary symptoms caused by chronic pain (e.g., not using certain parts of the body).

The chronic pain market is huge and is an active area of research. New drugs are being approved every day.

The benefits you can obtain from good self-management may outweigh and be longer-lasting than the benefits from drugs. A drug is considered effective and is approved for use if the drug leads to at least a 30% decrease in pain and if this decrease is statistically greater in the group receiving the active drug than in the group receiving a placebo (sugar pill). In some cases, the difference in efficacy between drugs and placebo is as little as 15%. Therefore, drugs are not a panacea.

Although medications may seem like a quick fix, here are some things to keep in mind if you and your physician are considering using pain medication:

- Medications do not cure or affect the causes of ME/CFS, FM or MCS. They act as a band-aid, allowing those who suffer from it some time and energy to develop more active strategies for pain management.
- All approved pain medications work well in the short term (e.g., 6-8 weeks). This is the necessary duration of use in studies required for regulatory approval. However, the long-term effectiveness of pain medications is much less clear. Virtually all classes of drugs lose effectiveness over time.
- Pain medications should NOT be used as a way to increase activity if this increase in activity has other adverse effects (e.g., causes an energy crash or cognitive dysfunction).
- In people with mild to moderate pain, pain medications can be used on an as-needed basis, but in people with severe pain, regular 24-hour use is necessary to prevent spikes of unbearable pain.
- Some medications can be easily used on an as-needed basis. This group includes anti-inflammatory drugs, muscle relaxants, and opiates. Other drugs, such as central desensitizers, need to be taken daily to work.

Anti-inflammatories: Non-steroidal anti-inflammatory drugs (NSAIDs) such as aspirin, naproxen, and ibuprofen are useful for inflammatory conditions such as arthritis. However, they are not very helpful in FM (chronic aching, burning, tiring muscle pain).

- If used over the long term, enteric-coated forms are preferred by most to minimize stomach problems. Even with the coating, many patients are unable to tolerate NSAIDS over the long term due to the side effect of stomach pain.
- The COX-2 inhibitor celecoxib (Celebrex®) is more specific in action than aspirin (ASA) and has fewer stomach side effects. However, like the other NSAIDS, COX-2 inhibitors are not very helpful for FM pain. The benefits may not outweigh the small increased risk of heart disease. It is because of this side effect that another COX-2 inhibitor, rofecoxib (Vioxx®), was taken off the market.
- If an NSAID helps, a *cardiac neutral* drug like naproxen is recommended.
- Be aware that all NSAIDS impact gut barrier integrity and can cause *leaky gut,* even if you don't notice symptoms of this.

Muscle Relaxants: For some people with FM, muscle spasm and myofascial pain are major problems.

- These people may benefit from the muscle relaxant cyclobenzaprine (Flexeril®). This can be used two to three times/day as needed, or at night to improve sleep. Cyclobenzaprine is related to the tricyclic antidepressants, and some patients do not tolerate the sedating or dry mouth side effects. Low-dose cyclobenzaprine (3 - 4 mg) was recently shown to be of use to improve EEG sleep profiles and decrease daytime fatigue and pain (see Session 2 for more on this).
- Muscle restlessness and pain associated with restless legs syndrome often respond to benzodiazepines such as clonazepam (Rivotril®) or diazepam (Valium®). These should be used with caution as all benzodiazepines are prone to tolerance (decreasing effects over time), withdrawal when stopped, and addiction in susceptible individuals.

Central Desensitizers: Several drugs initially designed for other purposes have shown benefit for some people with chronic pain, including FM pain. These drugs (unlike anti-inflammatories and pain killers) must be taken daily to be of benefit. They do not work minutes to hours after being taken, but only after they have been in the body at a sufficient concentration for several days to weeks. These drugs are not prone to misuse since there is no immediate beneficial effect. The more frequent problem is that patients forget to take the medication because the connection between taking the pill and the decrease in pain is delayed.

- The most commonly used centrally acting agent is amitriptyline (Elavil®). This is an older antidepressant that, in low doses, promotes sleep and decreases pain levels. Side effects include daytime sedation, constipation, and weight gain in some people.

- A number of anti-seizure medications are being used for chronic pain. The older agents, carbamazepine (Tegretol®) and valproate (Epival®), can decrease central pain and have prophylactic benefits for migraine sufferers. They are also mood stabilizers and are commonly used in psychiatry.
- Newer anti-seizure medications are also being used for pain management. The most commonly used drugs in this group are gabapentin (Neurontin®) and pregabalin (Lyrica®). My experience with gabapentin is that while it helps people who have neuropathic or nerve pain (e.g., diabetes), it is not very helpful for classical FM pain. Side effects include sleepiness and weight gain. Pregabalin is more helpful for FM pain, but the side effects of weight gain, cognitive dysfunction, and swelling of the limbs limit its use. Topiramate (Topamax®) is less studied in chronic pain but seems to be helpful in headache prophylaxis. Topiramate decreases rather than increases appetite. Again, remember that none of these drugs work quickly (i.e., the same day they are taken).
- Serotonin and Noradrenaline Reuptake Inhibitors (SNRIs) have recently been marketed for chronic pain and FM in particular. Venlafaxine (Effexor®) and duloxetine (Cymbalta®) are two SNRIs on the market in Canada. In my practice, venlafaxine has not proven to be at all effective for pain control. Duloxetine can be helpful for neuropathic and FM pain, but also has limiting side effects, including nausea and cognitive problems. If trying duloxetine, I recommend starting with a very low dose and gradually building to the usual therapeutic dose of 60 - 80 mg/day. There is more on antidepressants in Session 8.

Cannabinoid Drugs: This class of drugs is another recent addition to the market. They act on the cannabinoid receptors in the brain, decreasing the release of pain messages to brain neurons. The drugs contain delta-9-tetrahydrocannabinol (THC), the most active component in marijuana. Two brands: nabilone (Cesamet®) and dronabinol (Marinol®) are approved for use in Canada for neuropathic pain and for the nausea and vomiting associated with cancer chemotherapy. A few of my patients have tried these and, despite the claim that medicinal cannabinoids are not supposed to make people "high," these patients have reported some disconcerting cognitive effects. Again, others have had success by starting with a much lower dose than usual and working up slowly.

Tramadol: This unique drug has both opiate and antidepressant qualities. It has been approved for use in fibromyalgia at doses not exceeding 400mg per day. In my experience, it has mild pain effects; it takes the edge off with minimal side effects.

Topical Analgesics: Drugs taken orally are absorbed in the small intestine and are immediately carried by blood to the liver. The liver doesn't know that someone has taken the drug on purpose, and it immediately breaks the drug down to allow it to be excreted through the kidneys. The liver's job is to get rid of toxins. In this way, most drugs have to be given in at least twice the necessary dose to account for liver metabolism. Furthermore, the drug circulates in the blood to all parts of the body, not just the areas with pain. This distribution to the entire body causes many of the unwanted side effects of oral drugs.

Topical delivery through gels applied to the skin has some advantages. First, after being absorbed through the skin into the blood and tissues, these drugs bypass the liver metabolism. Secondly, since drugs are most active where they are applied, the effects on the rest of the body are much less.

There are, however, some limitations to using topical delivery of drugs. First, some drugs don't absorb well through the skin. They must be mixed with other substances to make them fat-soluble and absorbable. This makes topical agents greasy and messy. They often rub off on clothing and bedding before the full effect is realized. Secondly, patients can develop allergies to the nonmedicinal agents in topical analgesics, such as the emollients. Some drugs are delivered by a patch, and the adhesive used in medicated pain patches often causes allergies over time. Lastly, in terms of limitations, the cardinal symptom of FM is "pain all over." It is not feasible to rub topical analgesics everywhere on the body. For this reason, topical agents are most useful when applied to selected body areas with the worst pain.

- Topical NSAID cream (e.g., Pennsaid®) can be useful for FM and arthritis pain and has fewer systemic side effects than oral NSAIDS.
- Topical capsaicin (hot pepper), though touted by some as effective, has only meager evidence of long-term effect. As many as 1/3 of patients cannot tolerate the burning side effects on the skin.
- Other drugs, commonly used orally, can be compounded and made into a topical gel, including amitriptyline, gabapentin, and ketamine. In my limited experience, these topical applications can be very helpful as an adjunct to reduce the amount of oral medication required.

Opiates

The guidance on opiates has changed considerably since I published this manual in 2012. We now know that the slow-release opiate drugs like Oxycontin® that were supposed to be safe and effective are not.

Opiates have been used throughout history and are the most effective painkillers available for acute pain. They act on the opioid receptors in the brain. Activation of these receptors decreases pain signals. The pain signals are still produced, but perception is turned down. Although opiates are among the most useful pain drugs for acute pain (e.g., post-surgery), they have many limitations for chronic use.

- Opiates are addictive, and millions of people have suffered after being prescribed opiates.
- Opiates interact with the opiate receptors in ways that increase pain (Moseley & Butler, 2017). This can occur within hours of fast-acting opiate use and within weeks with chronic treatment (Lee, Silverman, Hansen, Patel, & Manchikanti, 2011).

- Opiates, once started, are hard to discontinue because decreasing the dose causes withdrawal symptoms. This is a physiological response and is not a sign of addiction or misuse. Withdrawal symptoms include increased pain. Thus, people are very resistant to decreasing the dose.
- Tolerance is almost universal with opiate use. This refers to the need over time to use an increased dose to achieve the same effect.
- Tolerance does not occur with the common opiate side effects such as severe constipation, nausea, itching, cognitive dysfunction, and sedation. They continue to plague users as long as they are taking the drug.
- Even with tolerance, the risk of death, if an opiate is accidentally or purposely taken in excess, is always present.
- It is difficult to travel if using opiates. A letter from your physician should suffice. However, since opiates are misused and abused, there is always the chance that possession will be misinterpreted as trafficking, resulting in seizure of the drugs and criminal charges, especially if crossing an international border.

For all these reasons, opiates should not be used in people with chronic pain. They don't work, may even make the pain worse and infer an unacceptable side effect risk.

Multidisciplinary Pain Clinics

Multidisciplinary pain clinics have the benefit of integrated care from clinicians from different fields, including physicians, psychologists, dietitians, and physiotherapists. Drawbacks include that most clinics are in larger cities, that wait times are long at some clinics, and that treatment is not individualized enough in some places.

A study of a 12-week multidisciplinary treatment program for FM showed a low percentage of responders. This is disappointing since many patients have huge hopes and expectations when attending a clinic with multiple professionals. The study conclusions were that current forms of treatment are not effective for a large portion of the FM population (King et al., 2002). This may change as discoveries are made.

Preparing for Session 8

Before reading the next session on depression and anxiety, it is strongly recommended that you spend 2 weeks focusing your attention on your mood and feelings. If you notice symptoms of depression, anxiety, anger, agitation, or other strong feelings, try to notice patterns so that you can determine if there are things that you could change. Your focus should be on noticing what makes these feelings better or worse.

You will need the following:

- Sleep Chart Adapted for Mood or Activity and Symptoms Chart.

Joan's Mood Chart

Joan decided to use the modified Sleep Chart (look for this in the Charts and Tools section). She knew that she had some problems with mood, but not with anxiety. She suspected that her mood might be related to her energy and her pain. Therefore, she decided to adapt the Sleep Chart to keep track of her mood, energy, and pain all at the same time.

During this charting period, Joan got the flu. This caused a spike in all of her symptoms, especially fatigue and pain. She was forced to miss a day of work and spent three days pretty much in bed or horizontal on the couch. She noticed that during this time, her mood dropped. Even when she recovered from the flu, her mood wasn't 10/10. She feels dragged down most days by her limitations. Pain and lack of energy prevent her from ever feeling really happy or content.

Name Joan Smith Date Feb 27/12 to Mar 11/12

Meds:

Supps: mood 10/10 = excellent 0/10 = horrible

Date	% Energy	Pain	Mood	Activities/other factors
Feb27	60	5	6	work 4 hours
28	55	5	5	visit father, more paperwork
29	60	6	6	errands, house work
Mar1	60	5	6	work 4 hours
2	50	4	7	lunch with friends yummy
3	35	7	5	got the flu - really crashed, pain ↑ — no dog walks ↓
4	30	8	4	in bed, ache all over
5	40	6	4	resting (missed work)
6	50	6	4	errands, groceries
7	55	5	5	visit parents - errands with mother
8	55	4	6	work 4 hours
9	50	5	6	rest
10	55	4	5	puttering, cooking.
11	60	6	6	church + park for walk ? perfume

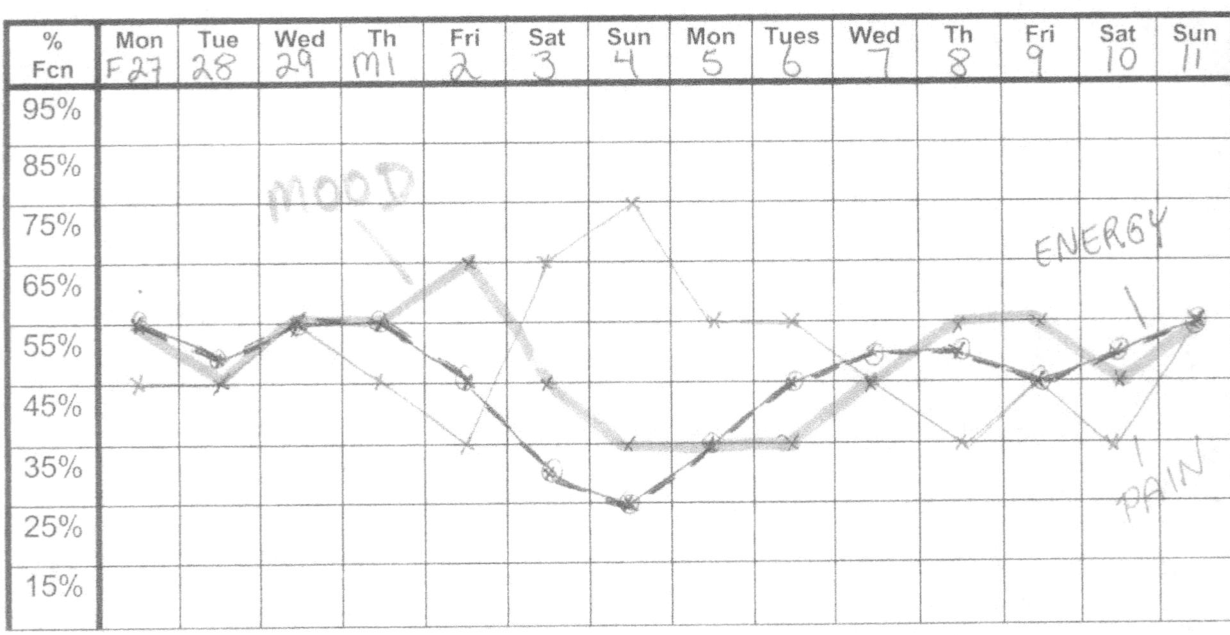

Adapted from the "sleep sheet" of Dr. Beverley Tompkins, Burke Institute, Calgary

Session 7 References

Adiguzel, O., Kaptanoglu, E., Turgut, B., & Nacitarhan, V. (2004). The possible effect of clinical recovery on regional cerebral blood flow deficits in fibromyalgia: a prospective study with semiquantitative SPECT. *South.Med.J*, 97, 651-655.

Bourne, E.J. (2001). *Anxiety and Phobia Workbook,* 3rd edn, pp. 1-436. New Harbinger Publications Inc., Oakland, California.

Bushnell, M.C., Villemure, C., Strigo, I., & Duncan, G.H. (2002). Imaging pain in the brain: The role of the cerebral cortex in pain perception and modulation. (Abstract).*J of Musculoskeletal Pain,* 10, 59-72.

Butler, D., Mosseley, L., & Sunyata (2003). *Explain Pain,* pp. 1-129. Noigroup Publications, Adelaide, Australia.

Cook, D.B., Stegner, A.J., & McLoughlin, M.J. (2007). Imaging pain of fibromyalgia. *Curr.Pain Headache Rep.*, 11, 190-200.

de Lange, F.P., Koers, A., Kalkman, J.S., Bleijenberg, G., Hagoort, P., van der Meer, J.W., & Toni, I. (2008). Increase in prefrontal cortical volume following cognitive behavioral therapy in patients with chronic fatigue syndrome. *Brain*, 131, 2172-2180.

Doidge, N. (2007). *The Brain that Changes Itself,* pp. 1-427. Penguin Books.

Giesecke, T., Gracely, R.H., Williams, D.A., Geisser, M.E., Petzke, F.W., & Clauw, D.J. (2005). The relationship between depression, clinical pain, and experimental pain in a chronic pain cohort. *Arthritis Rheum.*, 52, 1577-1584.

Gracely, R.H., Petzke, F., Wolf, J.M., & Clauw, D.J. (2002). Functional magnetic resonance imaging evidence of augmented pain processing in fibromyalgia. *Arthritis Rheum.*, 46, 1333-1343.

Graven-Nielsen, T., Aspegren, K.S., Henriksson, K.G., Bengtsson, M., Sorensen, J., Johnson, A., Gerdle, B., & Arendt-Nielsen, L. (2000). Ketamine reduces muscle pain, temporal summation, and referred pain in fibromyalgia patients. *Pain*, 85, 483-491.

Jeffers, S. (2007). *Feel the Fear and Do It Anyway,* pp. 1-240. Vermillion.

King, S.J., Wessel, J., Bhambhani, Y., Sholter, D., & Maksymowych, W. (2002). Predictors of success of intervention programs for persons with fibromyalgia. *J Rheumatol.*, 29, 1034-1040.

Lee, M., Silverman, S., Hansen, H., Patel, V., & Manchikanti, L. (2011). A Comprehensive Review of Opioid-Induced Hyperalgesia. *Pain Physician, 14*, 145–161. doi:https://dx.doi.org/10.36076/ppj.2011/14/145

Lutz, J., Jager, L., de, Q.D., Krauseneck, T., Padberg, F., Wichnalek, M., Beyer, A., Stahl, R., Zirngibl, B., Morhard, D., Reiser, M., & Schelling, G. (2008). White and gray matter abnormalities in the brain of patients with fibromyalgia: a diffusion-tensor and volumetric imaging study. *Arthritis Rheum.*, 58, 3960-3969.

May, A. (2008). Chronic pain may change the structure of the brain. *Pain*, 137, 7-15.

Moseley, G. L., & Butler, D. S. (2017). *Explain Pain Supercharged*. Adelaide, SA: NOIgroup Publications.

Nijs, J., Van de, P.K., Louckx, F., Truijen, S., & De, M.K. (2008). Exercise performance and chronic pain in chronic fatigue syndrome: the role of pain catastrophizing. *Pain Med.*, 9, 1164-1172.

Pall, M.L. & Satterlee, J.D. (2001). Elevated nitric oxide/peroxynitrite mechanism for the common etiology of Multiple Chemical Sensitivity, chronic fatigue syndrome, and posttraumatic stress disorder. *Annals of the New York Academy of Sciences*, 933.

Staud, R. (2010). Is it all central sensitization? Role of peripheral tissue nociception in chronic musculoskeletal pain. *Curr.Rheumatol.Rep.*, 12, 448-454.

Yunus, M.B. (2007). Fibromyalgia and overlapping disorders: the unifying concept of central sensitivity syndromes. *Semin.Arthritis Rheum.*, 36, 339-356.

Session 8

Depression and Anxiety

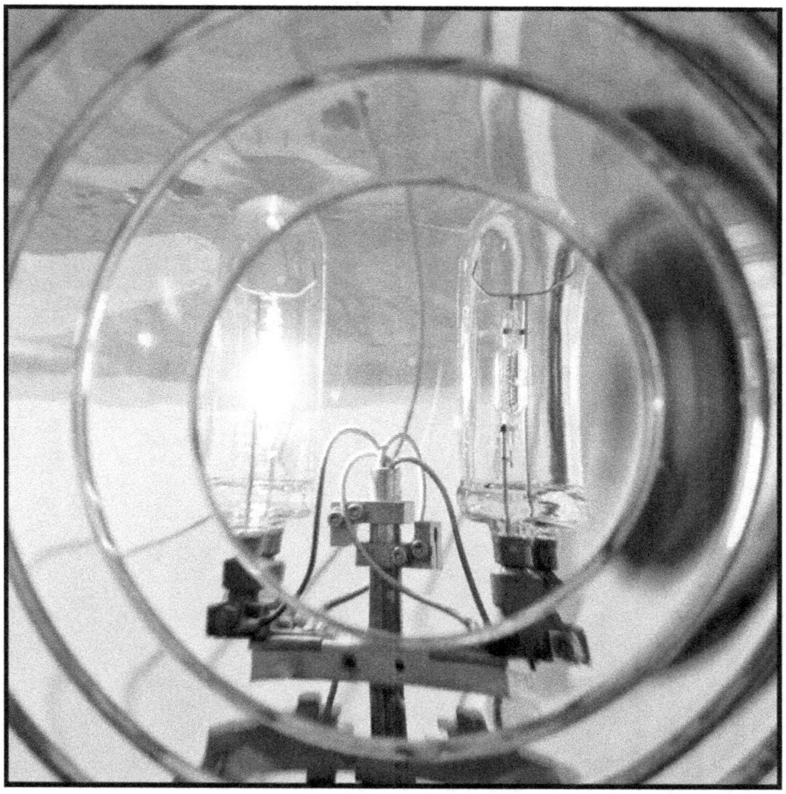

The Guiding Light

We are putting it all together.
There are still complexities, but our symptoms are bearable.
We are getting our lives back. We can see it now.
Our lives are different than before. We must never look back.
We must welcome our new lives. We must revel in our new future.
Acceptance is the key.
The light is on. This is our new reality.
I know it, I've done it.

The Road Well Traveled Part IV

Session 8

Depression and Anxiety

Objectives

- To understand more about the mind-body connection.
- To become familiar with some of the differences between ME/CFS, FM and MCS, and the psychiatric conditions: *major depression* and *generalized anxiety disorder*.
- To become familiar with common presentations of depression and anxiety in people with ME/CFS, FM and MCS.
- To understand the treatment strategies for depression and anxiety in people with ME/CFS, FM and MCS.

In this session, I use the terms *psychological symptoms* or *symptoms* to refer to feelings and ways of coping that detract from optimal health. Feelings of depression, anxiety, anger, and non-acceptance fit into this category. I use the terms *psychiatric disorder*, *disorder*, or *psychiatric condition* to refer to formal psychiatric conditions that are diagnosed and treated by psychiatrists. Examples of psychiatric disorders include autism, schizophrenia, obsessive-compulsive disorder, major depression, and generalized anxiety disorder.

The difference between depression (low mood), which is a common symptom experienced at times by almost everyone, and major depression, which is a psychiatric disorder, is that a diagnosis of major depression requires many criteria to be met in addition to low mood. Whereas the symptom of depression can come and go with life experiences, major depression is a group of symptoms present most days and is severe enough to cause disability.

This is similar to the difference between fatigue, a common symptom experienced by many people, and ME/CFS, a defined set of symptoms that occur together for a certain length of time and commonly cause disability. Thus, in this session, I refer to *depression* and *anxiety* as symptoms, and *major depression* and *generalized anxiety disorder* as disorders. The criteria for these latter two appear later in this session.

Why It Matters How We Classify a Condition

If you have done any reading on the topics of ME/CFS, FM and/or MCS, you will know that there is an active debate amongst researchers, clinicians, and patients about whether the cause and cure for these conditions are located in the mind or in the body. This debate is not unique to the fields of ME/CFS, FM or MCS. Similar debates have played out regarding conditions including scurvy, tuberculosis, asthma, and multiple sclerosis. In each of these latter cases, the debate was resolved when medical research found a biomedical cause for the condition.

In this section, I go into some detail about the debate about the classification of ME/CFS, FM and MCS because the treatments you are offered may depend on how your illness has been classified. As well, understanding the arguments on both sides may help you in negotiating medical or psychological care and in advocating with insurers or employers.

The placement of a condition on either the body or the mind end of the body-mind spectrum has important implications. It affects how society and medicine think about a disorder and which treatments are available or recommended. For example, no one would argue that cancer is a biomedical (body) condition; it is visible to the naked eye and even more clearly under a microscope. Without treatment, cancer grows. Tumors utilize the body's limited resources and cause many symptoms, including death. Psychological interventions are immensely helpful and often recommended to people suffering from cancer, but they do not take the place of biomedical treatments such as surgery and chemotherapy.

Major depression, on the other hand, is considered a psychiatric (mind) condition because the primary manifestation is psychological. The treatments of choice include antidepressant medication (drugs that act primarily on the brain) and psychotherapy (talk therapy) to help people evaluate their beliefs and gain perspective. However, exercise is also recommended for major depression because activating the body helps improve mood. Thus, treatments for major depression (many of which are often recommended for the symptom of depression) focus on the brain and/or the mind, but the body also has an important role to play.

It follows from this that if ME/CFS, FM and MCS are considered primarily as biomedical conditions, the primary treatments will be directed towards the body. If, on the other hand, they are considered primarily as psychiatric conditions, the treatments will be primarily directed at the brain and mind. For the record, based on reading the extensive medical literature on the topic and my clinical observations, and at the risk of further promoting polarization, I believe ME/CFS, FM and MCS to be primarily diseases of the body for which biological treatments are necessary for recovery. As with other conditions that are primarily biological, such as cancer, arthritis, and heart disease, interventions to help the mind and spirit are invaluable adjuncts but are rarely curative.

It is my belief that all symptoms, whether they seem to be physical or psychological in presentation, have a basis in biology at the cellular level. Neurotransmitters and inflammatory molecules move between the brain and the body (especially the gut), and most conditions are marked by a combination of "seemingly" physical and "seemingly" psychological symptoms. The bio-psycho-social model of disease that I talked about in Session 4 recognizes the interconnections. A compelling argument can be made that the distinction many of us draw between the mind and the body is artificial and that this artificial distinction has a negative effect on health outcomes. The current, often heated, debate about the correct understanding of ME/CFS in particular wouldn't be that important if it weren't for the important treatment implications that arise from what classification is chosen.

In the late 1980s, soon after ME/CFS was 're-discovered,' virtually all researchers assumed it to be a bio-medical condition triggered by infection. However, early research failed to find a single infectious cause. Frustrated researchers made the mistake of concluding that because no clear biomedical cause could be found, the condition must be psychological in origin. The following quote by then Toronto psychiatrists, Susan Abbey and Paul Garfinkel, is typical of this early change of heart about ME/CFS: "the majority of its sufferers are experiencing primary psychiatric disorders or psychophysiological reactions and the disorder is often a culturally sanctioned form of illness behavior" (Abbey & Garfinkel, 1991).

Despite the thousands of published peer-reviewed papers since the 1980s reporting abnormal biological findings in ME/CFS, FM and MCS that are different from findings in depression or any other psychiatric disorder, the "primarily psychiatric" view continues to have influence. In the absence of valid diagnostic tests, the fallback position seems to be that these conditions are essentially psychological. While few would argue with the importance of psychological factors, the dismissal of the biomedical contribution is of concern. For example, because of the NICE guidelines in the UK, some patients with ME/CFS are denied biomedical therapies and offered only cognitive behavioral therapy (CBT) or graded exercise therapy (GET) (Baker & Shaw, 2007). Hopefully, this misguided tendency is happening less since the newest NICE guidelines were published, explicitly recommending against graded exercise therapy (section 1.11.14 NICE Guidelines https://www.nice.org.uk/guidance/ng206/chapter/Recommendations).

More recently, the arguments for psychological causation have been cloaked in different terminology. It has been written that ME/CFS, FM, MCS and other conditions, such as irritable bowel syndrome and migraine headache, are *functional somatic syndromes* (Wessely et al., 1999). Historically, the term functional has been used to describe conditions that have no organic or physical/structural underpinning but are rather disturbances in the function of the cells or organs. Many of these so-called functional conditions, such as schizophrenia, are now firmly believed to reflect measurable changes in brain anatomy as well as function. Like the mind and the body, structure and function are closely tied.

The functional somatic syndrome terminology is difficult to argue with since it doesn't overtly state that the conditions mentioned are psychological in origin. However, interestingly, the authors who use this terminology are proponents of solely psychological interventions (Wessely et al., 1989). The rationale for using psychological interventions is the hypothesis that people with functional somatic syndromes hold faulty beliefs such as: "the belief that one has a serious disease; the expectation that one's condition is likely to worsen; the sick role, including the effects of litigation and compensation; and the alarming portrayal of the condition as catastrophic and disabling" (Barsky & Borus, 1999). These same authors also refer to the symptoms of ME/CFS, FM and MCS, among others, as "medically unexplained symptoms" or medically unexplained physical symptoms (MUPS). In my opinion, this is equally problematic (Aaron & Buchwald, 2001).

The mind/body debate is currently playing out in the Diagnostic and Statistical Manual V (DSM-5), the fifth iteration of the most commonly used psychiatric diagnostic manual in North America. New categories of simple somatic symptom disorder (SSSD) and complex somatic symptom disorder (CSSD) have been created. The criteria for the new categories, simple somatic symptom disorder and complex somatic symptom disorder, are problematic as they require the diagnosing physician to decide if a patient's symptoms are medically explained and/or worry about symptoms is excessive. Similar debates are also underway regarding the revision of the ICD (International Classification of Diseases) used outside North America.

The problem with these new criteria, like the concept of functional somatic syndrome before them, is that they assume that somatic (physical) symptoms must, if there is no medical explanation, be a reflection of psychological distress. This assumption fails to acknowledge that there is so much in medicine still unknown. It ignores the possibility that a biomedical explanation exists for which there is, as yet, no test or evidence. For example, some patients could have severe symptoms and be worried, but a test doesn't exist to validate whether their experience is true, false, or otherwise.

The new categories were included in DSM-5 and, as predicted, are being used in ways that minimize and invalidate the experiences of people with complex chronic conditions.

Sadly, for those with ME/CFS, FM and MCS, much time and energy is taken up with this semantic argument and not enough with research into causes and treatments of these common, disabling conditions.

While not strictly related to the classification of the conditions, the status of ME/CFS, FM and MCS as "contested conditions" has an impact on treatment as well. Contested conditions are those in which the aetiology (cause), diagnostic criteria, or prevalence are matters of controversy. As explained in Session 1, there is no gold-standard test for diagnosing ME/CFS, FM or MCS. Physicians must first rule out other conditions before applying the diagnostic criteria.

Patients with contested illness face many issues, including not being believed by family, friends, and/or health care professionals; not being able to access appropriate treatment; and not being able to access needed social and in-home support. Patients report that this lack of validation has a significant impact on them (Swoboda, 2008; Asbring & Narvanen, 2003).

How ME/CFS, FM and MCS Differ From Known Psychiatric Disorders

This section explains some of the differences between ME/CFS and FM and the psychiatric conditions with which they can most easily be confused: major depression and generalized anxiety disorder. Where the evidence is available for MCS, I have included it as well. As noted at the outset of this session, depression and anxiety can appear as feelings (symptoms) without a diagnosable psychiatric condition being present.

Rates of Psychiatric Disorder in ME/CFS, FM and MCS

If ME/CFS, FM and MCS were psychiatric disorders, symptoms such as depression, anxiety, hallucinations, or obsessions should be present in 100% of patients. While rates of psychiatric diagnosis in people with these conditions are high, they are not 100%. There is quite a bit of variation in the rate of psychiatric diagnosis amongst studies. Many early studies did find high rates of psychiatric symptoms in patients with ME/CFS and FM (Wessely et al., 1996; Manu et al., 1993).

These studies were conducted in tertiary care populations—patients attending a university clinic. University clinic patients are known to be more severely ill and to have more complicated conditions than the average patient attending his/ her/ their family physician, or people who have symptoms but never sought care.

When studies were done using general population samples, the prevalence of known psychiatric disorders among patients with ME/CFS was similar to the rates in patients with other chronic, disabling medical conditions, such as rheumatoid arthritis; approximately 40 - 60% (Nater et al., 2009; Axe & Satz, 2001). This implies that there is nothing special or different between ME/CFS and other medical conditions in terms of psychiatric factors.

The situation of FM is a bit more complicated. Rates of depression and anxiety are high in FM (Thieme et al., 2004). In addition, there seems to be some overlap in the genetics and family clustering of FM and depression, something not found in ME/CFS (Arnold et al., 2004a). Family clusters suggest a possible genetic overlap between FM and Major Depression. It is also thought that the presence of depression augments pain perception and is associated with a poorer outcome (Aguglia et al., 2010).

Despite all of this, in a recent review of the connection between FM and depression, Pae and colleagues conclude: "Our findings point to substantial similarities in neuroendocrine abnormalities, psychological characteristics, physical symptoms, and treatments between FM and major depressive disorder.

Despite overlap, the available findings do not support the assumption that major depressive disorder and FM refer to the same underlying construct or can be seen as subsidiaries of one disease concept" (Pae et al., 2008). Treatment with duloxetine (Cymbalta®), a drug with antidepressant and anti-pain properties, has independent effects on mood and pain. This adds to the evidence that although FM and depression are related, they are not the same condition (Arnold et al., 2005).

There is very little research directly on the intersection between MCS and psychiatry. There are a few small studies, but no large epidemiological studies as exist with ME/CFS and FM (Fiedler et al., 1996) (Simon et al., 1990; Caccappolo-van Vliet et al., 2002). The prevalence of psychiatric disorder in MCS seems to be elevated, but far from present in 100% of patients.

The prevalence of psychiatric disorders reported in studies varies considerably based on how it is measured. In one German study using a computerized instrument (known to be problematic for overestimating rates of psychiatric disorders in medical patients), 81% of patients with MCS were found to have a psychiatric diagnosis (Dietel et al., 2006). Another study, also German, which used a different methodology, found the rate to be 39% (Bornschein et al., 2002). The remainder of this section summarizes the literature about the relationship of ME/CFS, FM and MCS to psychiatric disorders, including studies only on ME/CFS and FM, since there is no more specific research on MCS.

Personality

Personality disorders are categorized as psychiatric conditions. These disorders begin early in life and are manifested by pervasive, inflexible, and counterproductive behavior patterns, especially patterns that annoy others. Personality disorders are strongly related to genetics and to early childhood experiences. They are much more common in patients with psychiatric conditions than in individuals without psychiatric symptoms. If ME/CFS or FM were primarily psychiatric conditions, one would expect that rates of personality disorder would be as elevated as they are in psychiatric samples. However, people with ME/CFS have similar rates of personality disorder (approximately 10%) as the general population and much lower rates than are found in patients with depression (Courjaret et al., 2009; Nater et al., 2010).

Genetics

Studies of large family groups suggest that there is some overlapping genetic predisposition in FM and depression. However, in ME/CFS, the common genetic profiles are quite different from those in depression. Furthermore, there are differences between the gene profiles found in people with ME/CFS when compared to FM. As well, the genetics of people with ME/CFS and FM who experienced mild to moderate symptom severity differed from the group with the most severe symptoms (Garcia-Fructuoso et al., 2008).

Predictors of Outcome

If ME/CFS were a psychiatric disorder, one would expect the presence and severity of psychological symptoms to predict outcome. However, this is not the case. Studies consistently show that symptom severity at onset and whether one meets full criteria for CFS predict prognosis in ME/CFS, but psychological symptoms and cognitive beliefs do not (Jones et al., 2004). Furthermore, in a Japanese study, the presence of a psychiatric disorder had no impact on the outcome in ME/CFS (Matsuda et al., 2009). In FM, the situation is different; the presence of depression is associated with a worse outcome in FM (Aguglia et al., 2010).

Connection Between Pain and Depression

Up to 65% of patients with depression experience pain, and up to 61% of chronic pain patients suffer from depression (Zheng et al., 2022). It has been unclear why this connection is so strong. Do people with chronic pain have pain because of depression, or experience depression because of their pain? I had believed that the direction of causality was primarily that having chronic pain is very stressful and leads to secondary depression.

It is now known that the neural circuits of pain and depression overlap (Moskowitz & Golden, 2013). This means that if one develops chronic pain, there is a likelihood of developing depression and vice versa, not only because of life circumstances but also because of overlap in how pain and emotions are processed in the brain. A recent analysis confirms that, although they share brain real estate, pain and depression are not exactly the same (Zheng et al., 2022). The brain areas connected with pain in the context of depression are different than those connected with depression in the context of pain. So, which condition came first seems to matter. This means it is worth giving priority to the condition that is primary and came first.

Connection Between ME/CFS, FM, Childhood Abuse and Anxiety Disorders

There is a higher rate of anxiety, including PTSD (post-traumatic stress disorder) and OCD (obsessive compulsive disorder), in people with ME/CFS and FM than in healthy individuals (Fischler et al., 1997). Childhood trauma, including abuse, increases the risk of anxiety disorders in adulthood, especially PTSD. It has been found that a history of childhood sexual abuse increases the risk of anxiety disorders in patients with ME/CFS, but doesn't predispose them to ME/CFS itself (Taylor & Jason, 2001). Some have suggested a causal link between childhood abuse and FM, but careful analysis of the data does not support this link (Raphael et al., 2006).

Joan's Mood Chart

Look at Joan's Mood Chart and your own for the discussion that follows. As mentioned in Session 7, Joan decided to use a modified Sleep Chart to observe if there were connections between her mood and other symptoms. She charted her mood, energy, and pain **all at the same time** for 2 weeks. During this charting period, Joan got the flu and noticed that her mood dropped. Even when she recovered from the flu, her mood wasn't 10/10. She feels dragged down most days by her limitations. Pain and lack of energy prevent her from ever feeling really happy or content.

You can see on Joan's Sleep Chart from Session 7 that her mood generally runs in parallel to her energy and inversely with her pain levels. However, there is a delay of a day or so between changes in Joan's energy and changes in her mood. This may suggest that Joan's mood changes are in reaction to her energy levels rather than a cause. It is hard to tell from this chart whether pain is causal in the shift of energy and mood. More charting of pain, together with the other symptoms, is required to see whether there is a pattern as to which symptoms change first and which follow. If Joan can identify this "lead symptom" (the one that precedes the others), then she should make it a focus of her self-management. If she can improve the lead symptom, the others may also improve.

Did you notice any connections between your mood, your energy, and/or your pain? Do you have a lead symptom on which you should be concentrating?

Subtypes of Psychological Symptoms Seen in Chronic Medical Conditions

Since symptoms of depression and anxiety are common in ME/CFS, FM and MCS, it is important to identify and manage these along with other symptoms. Just as with sleep, pain, diet, and avoidance of chemical toxins, if severe psychological symptoms are not managed, they are likely to impair the ability to function and regain health. In my practice, the severity of psychological symptoms ranged from very mild to very severe. I saw the full spectrum of psychological and psychiatric conditions amongst my patients with ME/CFS, FM and MCS. Patients with these conditions come from all walks of life, with a wide variety of childhood, family, and cultural backgrounds.

Just like people without physical health challenges, some people with ME/CFS, FM and MCS are psychologically robust and manage well in the face of significant stressors and severe health conditions. Others are vulnerable to psychological symptoms, and their thinking and feelings impact their daily functioning. In trying to figure out who needs psychological support and how to best give that support, I have developed the following five categories to subtype psychological symptoms in the context of chronic physical illness. These categories guide the types of recommendations I give to my patients with ME/CFS, FM and MCS who also suffer from psychological symptoms.

1. Grief

Grief is a common reaction of patients with all serious chronic health conditions, and I deal at some length with it in Session 4. It occurs in reaction to loss of health, social connections, family support, financial capability, career, and uncertainty regarding all of these. Grief itself is considered a normal reaction to tragedy and is not a psychiatric condition unless it is so severe that it impairs function or lasts beyond a time considered "normal." In chronic conditions that wax and wane, grief can be long-lived since new losses can accumulate and change. If the grief becomes so severe that it prevents people from looking after themselves and their health, then it may be considered a form of depression. This is often referred to as reactive or secondary depression since the loss of hope is secondary to the physical condition and the losses stemming from chronic ill health. When using the Sleep Chart to note mood, grief follows a path that parallels life stressors more than other symptoms. For example, if one gets bad news or develops a new health symptom, grief may worsen.

2. Worry

Worry about health, including prognosis, cause of symptoms, or unpredictability of symptoms, is common among people with chronic conditions. The status of ME/CFS, FM and MCS as *contested conditions* means that patients with these conditions are likely to have been ill for many years and seen many health care professionals before getting a diagnosis.

Lack of validation and support can feed worry about the nature of their condition (i.e., is it really FM or something "more serious"). This type of anxiety is made worse by dismissive health care professionals who don't take the time to explain why they believe a certain test or diagnosis is not a good fit, and by professionals who are not adequately educated about these conditions and cannot answer critical questions.

Worry from the impact of having ME/CFS, FM or MCS (e.g., loss of social connections, loss of family support, financial hardship, and loss of career) is also common. Financial worry results from the inability to work and the difficulty in getting and keeping disability support. Patients with ME/CFS (44%), FM (43%) and MCS (34%) are at high risk of poverty, defined as living on an annual income of less than CAD $ 15,000 (Parlor, 2009). This is a significant cause of anxiety in my patients.

3. Psychological Symptoms That Are Part of the Condition (i.e., biologically caused)

The same biological changes that cause physical symptoms can affect mood. Immune chemicals such as the cytokine IL-6 are known to be associated with ME/CFS and major depressive disorder. With "biologically caused psychological symptoms," one notices that the psychological and physical symptoms parallel each other on the Sleep Chart. This type of symptom is seen in other chronic neurological conditions, such as Parkinson's Disease and multiple sclerosis, where the brain itself is affected and both body and mind develop symptoms.

4. Comorbid Psychological Symptoms

As mentioned above, psychological symptoms can occur independent of, or at the same time as, ME/CFS, FM or MCS. This would be a case of really bad luck to have two or more serious conditions (comorbid). Comorbid conditions would be suspected if a patient had a history of psychological or psychiatric problems before the onset of the physical condition, or if the physical and psychological symptoms do not seem related to each other when graphing.

5. Substance-Induced Psychological Symptoms

Mood, anxiety, irritation, anger, and other symptoms can be triggered or worsened by medication or food, or withdrawal from either of these. People often forget that foods have drug-like properties. Some foods or food additives cause psychological reactions just as they cause physical reactions. As was discussed in Session 5, food also influences the bacteria that grow in the colon, and these bacteria produce chemicals that can influence psychological well-being.

Diagnosing Major Depression

NOTE: Making a psychiatric diagnosis should be undertaken by a physician, ideally a psychiatrist. Self-diagnosis is fraught with risk. Symptoms from many disorders overlap and can be confusing. This section and the next one on diagnosing generalized anxiety disorders are provided so that you are aware of the criteria used for diagnosing these two conditions. It does not take the place of expert advice.

The psychiatric disorder major depression includes in the list of diagnostic criteria (see below) some symptoms such as disrupted sleep, decrease in energy, and cognitive problems, which also occur commonly in ME/CFS, FM and MCS. If physicians don't ask about ALL the symptoms of each disorder, including the ones that do not commonly occur in ME/CFS, FM and MCS, they are at risk of making an incorrect diagnosis. Leonard Jason's group at De Paul University in Chicago has found that psychiatric conditions are often missed in patients with ME/CFS (Torres-Harding et al., 2002).

The chart below explains some of the overlap and differences between ME/CFS and major depression. With this information, it is relatively easy to discriminate between ME/CFS and major depression. It is more difficult to differentiate between fibromyalgia and major depression because the diagnostic criteria for FM are so nonspecific.

Clinicians must rely more on clinical judgment to determine which symptoms came first and which are more clinically relevant. MCS is fairly easy to differentiate from all other conditions since the symptoms are clearly related to chemical exposures and fluctuate considerably from day to day. Psychiatric disorders are present for most of the day, every day.

You May Have Major Depression if

- The depressive symptoms started before the physical disorder.
- Pessimism and lack of hope are generalized beyond health and illness-related issues.
- You are stuck in daily severe depression, and it is having a negative effect on your ability to manage your health condition and life.

ME/CFS	Major Depression
Clinical Presentation	
Infectious onset in the majority of cases	Rarely follows infectious illness
Fatigue is necessary for diagnosis	Mood change is necessary for diagnosis
Muscle and/or joint pain and significant headaches	Not usually associated with pain symptoms
Afternoon and evening are usually the worst times of day	Morning is usually the worst time of day
Orthostatic intolerance, tachycardia, and other autonomic dysfunctions are common	No association with autonomic symptoms
Immune manifestations, including tender lymph nodes, sore throat, chemical and food sensitivities	No association with immune symptoms
Loss of temperature stability and intolerance to extremes of temperature	No association with temperature problems
Fatigue and other symptoms are worsened by physical or mental exercise	Fatigue and mood improve with exercise
Decreased positive affect (energy, enthusiasm, happiness)	Increased negative affect (apathy, hopelessness, suicidal ideation, self-reproach)
Children have a better prognosis than adults	Children have a worse prognosis than adults

Diagnostic Criteria for Major Depression

Based on the DSM-IV-R (the current version of the Diagnostic and Statistical Manual used in psychiatry), to qualify for a diagnosis of major depression, you must meet the following criteria:

5 or more of the following symptoms:

1. Depressed mood (sad or empty) most of the day, nearly every day.
2. Decreased interest or pleasure in most activities nearly all the time.
3. Significant (>5% change) weight loss or weight gain not due to dieting and/or change in appetite (up or down).
4. Insomnia or hypersomnia (oversleeping) nearly every day.
5. Objective (notable by others) psychomotor agitation/retardation nearly all the time.
6. Fatigue or loss of energy nearly every day.
7. Feelings of worthlessness or excessive guilt nearly every day.
8. Decreased ability to think or concentrate, or indecisiveness, nearly every day.

Plus, the following:

- Duration of > 2 weeks
- Level of functioning decreased from before
- Must have either depressed mood or loss of interest or pleasure

The last criterion, "must have either depressed mood or loss of interest or pleasure," excludes patients with physical symptoms, but no depressed mood or loss of pleasure in life, from being classified as depressed. According to DSM-IV-R, if the subject has only physical symptoms (i.e., items 3, 4, 5, 6, 8 only), a diagnosis of depression cannot be made. Depression of mood must be present. If the patient has symptoms 3, 4, 5, 6, 8 AND has at least one of items 1, 2 or 7, then the criteria are met, and a diagnosis of major depression is valid. Ask yourself which activities you enjoy when you feel well or better. If you can't think of anything, consider depression.

As I've already noted, making a psychiatric diagnosis should be undertaken with a physician, ideally a psychiatrist. You can assist your physician by keeping careful track of your psychological symptoms. The visual graph at the bottom of the Sleep Chart can be very useful in making the connection, or lack thereof, between psychological symptoms and your other symptoms. To determine if your physical and psychological symptoms are connected (e.g., biologically caused symptoms), ask yourself: "Do I often have a good day with respect to energy but a bad day with respect to mood?" If the answer is "yes," then the mood disorder is independent of your physical condition.

Having an independent mood disorder is relatively good news (if you must be depressed at all) because these types of depression (whether depressive symptoms or meeting full criteria for major depressive disorder) are easier to treat than a depression that is an inherent part of the ME/CFS, FM or MCS. If your psychological symptoms parallel your physical symptoms, it may mean that depression or anxiety is part of your ME/CFS, FM or MCS (i.e., biologically caused). This is the most challenging type of psychological symptom to treat. It doesn't usually respond to common drug or psychotherapy treatments. To get relief from these parallel symptoms may require recovery or significant improvement from the ME/CFS, FM or MCS.

Don't forget ...

When trying to make a diagnosis, the following core symptoms must be present:

- The necessary symptom for making a diagnosis of clinical depression is a persistent low or irritable mood, and/or anhedonia (not feeling any pleasure), guilt, or self-blame.
- The necessary symptom for making a diagnosis of ME/CFS is post-exertional malaise lasting more than 24 hours. The additional symptoms outlined in Session 1 must also be present. Those who think of ME/CFS as "fatigue" and forget the importance of the other symptoms will risk misdiagnosis and inappropriate treatment recommendations.
- The necessary symptom for making a diagnosis of FM is pain all over. Those who think that FM is "masked depression" will overestimate the presence of depression and may ignore other useful management strategies.
- The necessary symptom for MCS is a reaction to chemical exposures, which then lessens with time after the exposure ceases.

Diagnosing Generalized Anxiety Disorder

NOTE: As indicated in the previous section, self-diagnosis is fraught with risk. This information does not take the place of expert advice.

You May Have an Anxiety Disorder if

- The anxiety started before the onset of the ME/CFS, FM or MCS.
- Anxiety is generalized and not limited to health and health care-related issues.
- You are unable to cope with or resolve anxiety over the long term.

Diagnostic Criteria for Generalized Anxiety Disorder (GAD)

Based on the 4th (current) version of the Diagnostic and Statistical Manual used in psychiatry (DSM-IV-R) to qualify for a diagnosis of generalized anxiety disorder, you must meet the following criteria:

1. Excessive worry on most days (about many things, not just illness).
2. Duration > 6 months.
3. Difficulty controlling worry.
4. Must have three or more of the following symptoms:
   - Feeling restless or keyed up
   - Easily fatigued
   - Difficulty concentrating/mind going blank
   - Irritability
   - Muscle tension
   - Sleep disturbance (difficulty falling asleep or unrefreshing sleep)
5. Symptoms cause clinically significant distress/impairment.
6. Symptoms are NOT due to direct physiological effects of a medical condition (e.g., ME/CFS).

Most patients with ME/CFS, FM or MCS will have three or more of the physical symptoms listed in category 4 of the above diagnostic criteria. Many are worried about their health and related problems. However, most will not be excessively worried about life every day and/or have difficulty controlling their worry. Most patients are able to put their worries aside for periods of time and focus on other aspects of life. If you **do not** have items 1, 3 and 6, you do not meet the criteria for generalized anxiety disorder. Other anxiety disorders, such as panic disorder, obsessive-compulsive disorder, and post-traumatic stress disorder, require anxiety to be present most of the time and to be interfering substantially with daily function.

Management of Psychological Reactions to ME/CFS, FM and MCS

In the case of patients who are suffering from grief or depression in reaction to their illness or their life situation, the best antidepressant is improved physical health. Validation of illness and life circumstances from professionals is very important. Patients tell me that feeling believed and taken seriously, even if I do not know how to help them get better, is helpful.

For patients who worry about their physician missing some other serious condition, having a health care professional take the time to explain why certain diagnoses may or may not be relevant is critical. It may be necessary to have tests or consultations to rule out feared diagnoses such as cancer, MS, or heart disease. Have a discussion with your physician about why this may or may not be useful in your case. Sometimes, no tests are needed. Be ready to accept this possibility if the reasons for it are explained to you adequately.

As with chronic pain, an active approach is necessary to manage depression and worry. A good starting point is appropriate self-management (e.g., ensuring adequate sleep, adequate diet, and adequate rest), as you have learned by working through this manual. If you don't attend to these critical aspects of your health, depression and worry are unlikely to improve. Treatment of physical symptoms such as low blood pressure, high heart rate, low blood sugar, irritable bladder and bowel is also helpful in easing grief and worry. Here is where the mind-body connection is important. You need to manage the mind to treat the body and vice versa.

To resolve suffering from grief, depression or worry about your situation, you may need to seek professional advocacy to obtain sustainable school/work conditions, leave of absence from school or work, or disability insurance, etc.

Then there is the most powerful of all remedies—time. It takes time to understand your health condition and learn what makes you feel as well as possible. It also takes time to work through the psychological trauma of having developed a little-understood condition, for which there is no cure. In my experience, most patients take several years to move through the stages of accepting and adapting to chronic illness. Some, especially those who struggle to face the reality of their situation, take longer.

Be patient with yourself. Give yourself time and have faith that with a bit of work on your part and access to accurate information (such as in this manual), you will begin to feel better emotionally. Review Session 4 (Coping with Chronic Illness), particularly the section on grief, for more ideas and self-reflective questions that may help you move through your grief, depression, or worry. Read other books on grief or chronic illness to get more ideas. As discussed in Session 4, everyone's path is unique. There is no recipe for success; you must follow your own intuition and do what seems right for you.

If, while you are on the path of recovery, you notice suicidal ideation, you should seek professional help. As in other serious chronic health conditions, suicide is an often-considered way of solving seemingly unsolvable problems. Suicide is one of the top three causes of death among patients with ME/CFS (Jason et al., 2006). Suicide rates are also increased among people with FM (Wolfe et al., 2011). As far as I am aware, suicide has not been studied in MCS.

If you are struggling, please get help. Supportive counselling and psychotherapy regarding health, career, peer group, and family issues can be extremely helpful. If you are feeling lost and overwhelmed, talking with a professional can help you gain perspective and formulate a new plan for your life. Men are much less likely to go for help than women. Don't be too proud to get the help you need. In my opinion, it is a strength and not a weakness to have the courage to talk about a situation openly with another person. Review the suggestions in Session 4 about whether psychotherapy is for you.

Treatment of Comorbid Psychiatric Disorders in ME/CFS, FM & MCS

When to Seek Professional Help

Comorbid means that you have a psychiatric condition and at the same time suffer from ME/CFS, FM or MCS. When to seek treatment depends on how serious the symptoms are and how much they are impairing your ability to live well. Treatment should be sought when hopelessness, pessimism, or worry impair your ability to maintain optimal self-management and impair your enjoyment of life. ME/CFS, FM and MCS are relentless conditions requiring daily management.

If you lose hope and feel you have nothing to look forward to, self-management won't be the priority it needs to be. This creates a vicious circle in which you don't attend to your self-care. Then health suffers, and depression and worry are reinforced, and you say to yourself, "You see, I knew it was hopeless."

Worrying, needless or not, is exhausting and to be avoided in people who already have energy limitations. Patients with anxiety disorders, in addition to ME/CFS, FM and MCS really suffer since anxiety doesn't take a break. Worry (the primary symptom of anxiety disorders) is maintained by the belief that if one worries enough, solutions (sometimes to insolvable problems) will be found.

- Do you have the belief that worrying will help you solve your problems?
- Do you fear that if you stop worrying, you will never solve your problems?
- Can you take even a few minutes or a few hours break from the worry?
- If so, think of the last time that worry led to a good outcome for you. Was the amount of worry expended worth the outcome?
- Do you want to continue to approach your life in this way, or are you ready for a change?

If you are ready for change, keep reading the rest of this section regarding resources for tackling anxiety problems.

Treatment of comorbid depression and anxiety is similar to treatment of these psychiatric conditions in the absence of a medical condition. Therefore, most mental health professionals should be able to help with this type of problem. First-line treatment for most types of depression and anxiety is a combination of medication and psychotherapy.

There are some characteristics of patients with ME/CFS, FM and MCS that influence the choice of treatment for comorbid psychiatric conditions. For example, severely ill patients may not have the physical or mental stamina to be able to benefit from psychotherapy of any kind. Many of my patients do not have the physical energy or cognitive function to attend and benefit from intensive therapy programs that are helpful for healthy individuals.

Sometimes programs are offered first thing in the morning, and though otherwise excellent, are inappropriate for patients who "don't do mornings." Treatment programs often lack the awareness that the energy limitations of patients with ME/CFS, FM and the inability to tolerate exposure to chemicals at a clinic are genuine and not due to poor motivation. Lack of understanding of patients' real limitations can lead to patients being blacklisted from mental health programs for seeming "non-compliant."

I recommend being upfront with service providers from the start rather than being optimistic. For example, if you are only able to leave the house twice per week (e.g., for groceries and church), don't commit to a weekly therapy program that you are unlikely to be able to maintain. It's always better to slightly underestimate your abilities and be successful than to overestimate and fail to complete a course of therapy. Remember the section on Goal Setting in Session 1?

More flexible mental health services are generally available privately, but many patients cannot afford to pay private rates. In the absence of having private insurance, some patients may not be able to access needed, even life-saving services.

Cognitive Behavior Therapy (CBT)

CBT is a mainstay of therapy for most types of depression and anxiety. This type of therapy is relatively acceptable to patients and useful to most people, even those who don't really want to dig deeply into emotional issues. To learn more about managing low mood, I recommend for depression Dr. David Burns' book *Feeling Good: The New Mood Therapy* (Burns, 2000). I mentioned this book (and more about CBT) in Session 4 in the section dealing with the cognitive-behavioral model. If your problem is primarily with anxiety, the *Anxiety and Phobia Workbook* is an excellent introduction to the common types of anxiety (Bourne, 2001). This book was already mentioned in Session 7 as a recommendation for people whose anxiety is worsening their pain. Both of these books also discuss medication treatments.

With a better understanding of your condition and the available treatments, you will be better equipped to find a suitable professional to help you along your path to better health. There are other types of therapy, and if CBT doesn't appeal to you, contact your local mental health service to see what other options are available. As mentioned in Session 4, if psychotherapy of any kind is used to convince patients with ME/CFS, FM and MCS that what they are experiencing is not real or serious, when in fact it is, it is disrespectful and inappropriate and not the type I am recommending here.

Antidepressant Drugs

Antidepressant drugs are the drugs of choice for both depression and anxiety. This is fortunate since many people suffer from symptoms of anxiety and depression at the same time. Antidepressant medication is indicated if symptoms of depression or anxiety are interfering with hope, sleep, and rehabilitation. For example, a person may be so hopeless that s/he doesn't have the motivation to make changes to their lifestyle that would improve pain and other symptoms.

Note that, though often used in people with ME/CFS, FM and MCS, antidepressant drugs do not improve the core symptoms of these conditions. However, since both depression and anxiety augment pain perception, the use of antidepressants decreases pain in some FM patients (Vercoulen et al., 1996; Arnold et al., 2007; Arnold et al., 2004b).

In ME/CFS, FM and MCS, antidepressants usually need to be started at lower doses than those tolerated by physically healthy patients. In some patients, with a gradual increase, usual therapeutic doses can be reached. With other patients, the full dose is not possible due to the severity of side effects. In some cases, even a lower-than-usual dose can be therapeutic. There is no research to prove this rule of thumb, but it is generally accepted in the field.

Some patients will be unable to tolerate any antidepressant. For these patients, there are a couple of non-pharmacological approaches that are worth trying. In my experience, drugs are more powerful and more effective than natural remedies. But natural remedies have a place if one is unable to tolerate any medication. Natural remedies can also be used to augment or strengthen the effect of antidepressants. Always consult your medical or naturopathic physician before adding any non-prescribed remedy to your management plan. Remember, natural is not synonymous with safe.

What follows is a summary of the natural and drug remedies for depression and anxiety that I find most effective and best tolerated by patients with ME/CFS, FM and MCS. Again, there is no research on drug choices, only clinical experience.

Eicosapentaenoic Acid (EPA): EPA is an omega-3 fatty acid found in fish oil. It has been used as a remedy for depression for many years, originally researched at Harvard University. A recent meta-analysis review of all the studies done to date shows that EPA is an effective treatment for major depression as long as EPA makes up more than 60% of the contents of each capsule and the dose of EPA in excess of DHA (the other fatty acid found in fish oil), ranges from 200 - 2000 mg (Sublette et al., 2011).

I find that the original Harvard guidelines of purified EPA capsules at a dose of at least eight capsules (4000mg) per day are effective. The brands OmegaBrite® and Omega+Joy® are two that meet purity and dose standards. Although a recent study reported that EPA was equally as effective as fluoxetine (Prozac®), I find that antidepressants are more effective (Jazayeri et al., 2008).

St. John's Wort: This herbal remedy has strong serotonin reuptake inhibitor (SSRI) properties. It is not surprising, therefore, that this remedy has been found to be equally effective as SSRI drugs in treating major depression (Linde et al., 2008; Rahimi et al., 2009). St. John's Wort is taken as a standardized 0.3% extract of hypericin 300 mg by mouth three times daily.

Because of its powerful effect on neurotransmitters, St. John's Wort has many side effects and a long list of drugs and other herbal supplements with which it can interact adversely. For safety, only use St. John's Wort under medical supervision and always tell your physician and pharmacist if you are taking it. In combination with other antidepressants or neurotransmitter precursors, the dangerous serotonin syndrome can occur.

Tricyclic Antidepressants: Low-dose tricyclic antidepressants such as amitriptyline (Elavil®), imipramine (Tofranil®), doxepin (Sinequan®) and others are often useful for sleep rehabilitation and pain management in FM, but rarely have antidepressant effects at the low doses used and tolerated by FM patients. The dose of tricyclics used in pain medicine ranges from 2 - 50 mg a day. The dose required for antidepressant effect ranges from 75 - 250 mg/day.

Neurotransmitter Reuptake Inhibitors: This drug family consists of most of the currently used antidepressants, including fluoxetine (Prozac®), citalopram (Celexa®), venlafaxine (Effexor®), and duloxetine (Cymbalta®). These drugs act by blocking the reuptake or recycling of either serotonin or noradrenaline at the nerve synapses in the brain. Blocking uptake leaves more of the transmitter in the synapse to bind to the receptors and augments the messages being passed from one nerve to the next. It is now commonly believed that depression, anxiety, and chronic pain are influenced by these neurotransmitter levels.

However, there is more to the story. The antidepressants bind to the majority of reuptake receptors within 24 hours, yet it takes 3-6 weeks for the antidepressant effect to occur and maximize. The therapeutic benefit likely arises as a result of the body's attempts to adapt to the changes caused by the drugs. These adaptations take several weeks to occur.

Comparison of Antidepressants

Until recently, it has been thought that all antidepressants have more or less the same efficacy. In 2009, a major meta-analysis of all of the studies directly comparing the newer antidepressants showed that, in fact, some drugs have a better track record than others (Cipriani et al., 2009). This comparison review was updated in 2018 to include recently introduced antidepressants (Cipriani et al., 2018).

This landmark study compared the effectiveness (does it work?) and acceptability (is it tolerated?) of 21 antidepressants commonly used for the treatment of major depressive disorder (MDD) in adults. The analysis included

- 522 double-blind randomized controlled trials including 116,477 participants published between 1979 and 2016.
- studies comparing the antidepressant drug to a placebo and to other drugs.

For the purposes of the analysis, an antidepressant was considered effective if there was a 50% or greater reduction on a depression scale score. Acceptability was determined by how many people dropped out of studies. Dropouts are most often due to ineffectiveness, side effects or a combination of both.

All 21 antidepressants studied were more effective than placebo. In the head-to-head comparisons, they found the following:

Best balance of effectiveness and acceptability

Escitalopram, Sertraline, Vortioxetine, Mirtazapine

This list contains three of the drugs found in the 2009 "best of" list: escitalopram (Lexapro®), sertraline (Zoloft®) and mirtazapine (Remeron®) and a new drug, vortioxetine (Trintellix® and Brintellix®). Vortioxetine was just being introduced in the past few years of my practice, and by anecdote seemed to live up to its selling feature of helping with cognitive function.

High effectiveness but lower tolerability

Paroxetine, Amitriptyline, Venlafaxine

I stopped prescribing paroxetine (Paxil®) when patients reported severe symptoms when they tried to stop the drug. I prescribed a lot of amitriptyline (Elavil®) and venlafaxine (Effexor®) in my complex chronic disease practice, and contrary to the Cipriani findings, I found both were generally effective and well tolerated in the ME community. Amitriptyline has many intolerable side effects when used at full antidepressant doses (200 – 300 mg), but when used at low doses (5 – 25 mg) for assistance with sleep and pain, it is often well tolerated and still has a mild antidepressant effect.

There are no studies on how well these drugs are tolerated in patients with ME/CFS, FM or MCS. I have learned the hard way that it is always better to start with 1/4 or 1/2 the normal starting dose and work up slowly. Many patients will be able to tolerate drugs given in this manner that they would react badly to if started in the usual way. Though safer, this slow approach means being even more patient for the drug to begin working since, even in sensitive patients, antidepressants generally need to be in the recommended dose range to be effective.

In choosing from the long list of available antidepressants, I prefer the drugs with a longer half-life. Half-life refers to the length of time it takes for 1/2 of the drug to be metabolized and excreted from the body. It is approximately equal to the duration of action.

- A drug with a half-life less than 12 hours generally needs to be taken 2-3 times per day to prevent peaks and valleys in symptom control.
- Drugs with longer half-lives can be taken once daily, which is more convenient and easier to remember.
- Drugs with longer half-lives are less likely to cause *discontinuation syndrome*, a very unpleasant syndrome of shooting pain, nausea, and other symptoms that can occur when trying to stop using an antidepressant.

As well, I prefer the drugs that act on both serotonin and noradrenaline since we do not yet have the tests to determine ahead of time which neurotransmitter is affected in a given individual. The drugs with multi-transmitter action include venlafaxine (Effexor®), duloxetine (Cymbalta®), bupropion (Wellbutrin®), and moclobemide (Manerix®, not on the above list).

In psychiatry, drugs are used not only for their beneficial effects but also to utilize side effects to advantage. For example, some antidepressants such as fluvoxamine (Luvox®) and mirtazapine (Remeron®) are very sedating and can be helpful in patients with sleep problems. Past history and family history also influence the choice of a drug. If you have had a good (or bad) response to a drug in the past, this is likely to occur again if you try the same drug. Similarly, if a close relative has had a good or bad experience on an antidepressant, this is important information for your physician to know.

If one drug doesn't work at full dose after a trial of 6-8 weeks, there are a number of strategies to try. If there is absolutely no response, your physician will likely try a drug with a different mechanism of action. If the first drug had some positive effect, the physician may choose to supplement the first drug with another drug. Common strategies for augmentation include adding a second antidepressant with a different mechanism of action, adding an atypical antipsychotic drug such as olanzapine (Zyprexa®) or quetiapine (Seroquel®), or adding lithium or T3 thyroid hormone. These strategies require an experienced family physician or consultation with a psychiatrist.

Benzodiazepines: This family of drugs includes diazepam (Valium®), alprazolam (Xanax®), lorazepam (Ativan®) and others. The benzodiazepines are the most effective drugs for anxiety. However, there are several drawbacks to their use.

- First, because benzodiazepines work right away (within 30 minutes of taking the pill), patients quickly develop psychological dependence on the drugs.

- People who use benzodiazepines on a regular basis develop physiological tolerance to the therapeutic effect and need a higher dose over time to achieve the same effect.
- When trying to stop a benzodiazepine drug after regular use, a discontinuation syndrome (including increased anxiety) occurs and can be very difficult to cope with.

For these reasons, the neurotransmitter reuptake inhibitors (listed above) are my preferred choice for anxiety. However, in certain circumstances, such as patients who have severe muscle tension or restless legs syndrome, a trial of the benzodiazepine clonazepam is indicated. This has a longer half-life and decreased tendency towards tolerance and addiction than the other benzodiazepines. However, people with anxiety find it less effective since it takes longer to work.

Preparing for Session 9

This is the end of Session 8. The next session, which provides some information about a number of commonly used treatments for one or more of ME/CFS, FM and MCS, does not require you to fill out a Chart, so you can proceed to it when you are ready. The suggestions in Session 9 are not self-management suggestions. They all require the assistance of a health care professional. They have been included in this manual so that you are aware of some of the commonly used (i.e., not experimental) treatments for these conditions. This is far from a complete list. The suggestions included are those that are the most mainstream (i.e., there is a good chance your health care professional will feel comfortable helping you with them) and most successful in my experience.

Session 8 References

Aaron, L.A. & Buchwald, D. (2001). A review of the evidence for overlap among unexplained clinical conditions. *Ann.Intern.Med.*, 134, 868-881.

Abbey, S.E. & Garfinkel, P.E. (1991). Neurasthenia and chronic fatigue syndrome: the role of culture in the making of a diagnosis. *American Journal of Psychiatry*, 148, 1638-1646.

Aguglia, A., Salvi, V., Maina, G., Rossetto, I., & Aguglia, E. (2010). Fibromyalgia syndrome and depressive symptoms: Comorbidity and clinical correlates. *J Affect. Disord.*

Arnold, L.M., Crofford, L.J., Martin, S.A., Young, J.P., & Sharma, U. (2007). The effect of anxiety and depression on improvements in pain in a randomized, controlled trial of pregabalin for treatment of fibromyalgia. *Pain Med.*, 8, 633-638.

Arnold, L.M., Hudson, J.I., Hess, E.V., Ware, A.E., Fritz, D.A., Auchenbach, M.B., Starck, L.O., & Keck, P.E., Jr. (2004a). Family study of fibromyalgia. *Arthritis Rheum.*, 50, 944-952.

Arnold, L.M., Lu, Y., Crofford, L.J., Wohlreich, M., Detke, M.J., Iyengar, S., & Goldstein, D.J. (2004b). A double-blind, multicenter trial comparing duloxetine with placebo in the treatment of fibromyalgia patients with or without major depressive disorder. *Arthritis Rheum.*, 50, 2974-2984.

Arnold, L.M., Rosen, A., Pritchett, Y.L., D'Souza, D.N., Goldstein, D.J., Iyengar, S., & Wernicke, J.F. (2005). A randomized, double-blind, placebo-controlled trial of duloxetine in the treatment of women with fibromyalgia with or without major depressive disorder. *Pain*, 119, 5-15.

Asbring, P. & Narvanen, A.L. (2003). Ideal versus reality: physicians perspectives on patients with chronic fatigue syndrome (CFS) and fibromyalgia. *Soc.Sci.Med.*, 57, 711-720.

Axe, E.K. & Satz, P. (2001). Depressive comorbidity in the fatiguing illnesses. Innovations in Chronic Fatigue Syndrome Research and Clinical Practice (ed. by R. Patarca-Montero), pp. 23-29. Haworth Medical Press, New York.

Barsky, A.J. & Borus, J.F. (1999). Functional somatic syndromes. *Annals of Internal Medicine*, 130, 910-921.

Bornschein, S., Hausteiner, C., Zilker, T., & Forstl, H. (2002). Psychiatric and somatic disorders and multiple chemical sensitivity (MCS) in 264 'environmental patients'. *Psychol.Med.*, 32, 1387-1394.

Bourne, E.J. (2001). *Anxiety and Phobia Workbook,* 3rd edn, pp. 1-436. New Harbinger Publications Inc., Oakland, California.

Burns, D. (2000). *Feeling Good: The New Mood Therapy,* pp. 1-706. Quill (Harper Collins), New York.

Buskila, D. & Cohen, H. (2007). Comorbidity of fibromyalgia and psychiatric disorders. *Curr.Pain Headache Rep.*, 11, 333-338.

Caccappolo-van Vliet, E., Kelly-McNeil, K., Natelson, B., Kipen, H., & Fiedler, N. (2002). Anxiety sensitivity and depression in Multiple Chemical Sensitivity and asthma. *J Occup. Environ.Med.*, 44, 890-901.

Cipriani, A., Furukawa, T.A., Salanti, G., Geddes, J.R., Higgins, J.P., Churchill, R., Watanabe, N., Nakagawa, A., Omori, I.M., McGuire, H., Tansella, M., & Barbui, C. (2009). Comparative efficacy and acceptability of 12 new-generation antidepressants: a multiple-treatments meta-analysis. *Lancet*, 373, 746-758.

Cipriani, A., Furukawa, T. A., Salanti, G., Chaimani, A., Atkinson, L. Z., Ogawa, Y., Leucht, S., Ruhe, H. G., Turner, E. H., Higgins, J. P. T., Egger, M., Takeshima, N., Hayasaka, Y., Imai, H., Shinohara, K., Tajika, A., Ioannidis, J. P. A., & Geddes, J. R. (2018). Comparative efficacy and acceptability of 21 antidepressant drugs for the acute treatment of adults with major depressive disorder: a systematic review and network meta-analysis. *The Lancet, 391*(10128), 1357–1366. https://doi.org/10.1016/S0140-6736(17)32802-7

Courjaret, J., Schotte, C.K., Wijnants, H., Moorkens, G., & Cosyns, P. (2009). Chronic fatigue syndrome and DSM-IV personality disorders. *J Psychosom.Res.*, 66, 13-20.

Dietel, A., Jordan, L., Muhlinghaus, T., Eikmann, T.F., Herr, C.E., Nowak, D., Pedrosa, G.F., Podoll, K., Wiesmuller, G.A., & Eis, D. (2006). Psychiatric disorders of environmental outpatients--results of the standardized psychiatric interview (CIDI) from the German multi-center study on Multiple Chemical Sensitivity (MCS). *Psychother.Psychosom.Med Psychol.*, 56, 162-171.

Fiedler, N., Kipen, H.M., DeLuca, J., Kelly-McNeil, K., & Natelson, B. (1996). A controlled comparison of Multiple Chemical Sensitivity and chronic fatigue syndrome. *Psychosomatic Medicine*, 58, 38-49.

Fischler, B., Cluydts, R., De, G.Y., Kaufman, L., & De, M.K. (1997). Generalized anxiety disorder in chronic fatigue syndrome. *Acta Psychiatr.Scand.*, 95, 405-413.

Garcia-Fructuoso, F., Lao-Villadoniga, J.I., Olano-Martin, E., Santos, C., Poca-Dias, V., Fernandez-Sola, J., Martinez, A., Simon, L., & Tejedor, D. (2008). Identification of differential genetic profiles in severe forms of fibromyalgia and chronic fatigue syndrome/myalgic encephalomyelitis: a population-based genetic association study. *Journal of Clinical Research*, 1, 1-25.

Jason, L.A., Corradi, K., Gress, S., Williams, S., & Torres-Harding, S. (2006). Causes of death among patients with chronic fatigue syndrome. *Health Care Women Int.*, 27, 615-626.

Jazayeri, S., Tehrani-Doost, M., Keshavarz, S.A., Hosseini, M., Djazayery, A., Amini, H., Jalali, M., & Peet, M. (2008). Comparison of therapeutic effects of omega-3 fatty acid eicosapentaenoic acid and fluoxetine, separately and in combination, in major depressive disorder. *Aust.N.Z.J Psychiatry*, 42, 192-198.

Jones, J., Hickie, I., Wakefield, D., Davenport, T.A., Vollmer-Conna, U., & Lloyd, A. (2004). The Dubbo Infection Outcomes Study: Post-infective Fatigue as a model for CFS.

Linde, K., Berner, M.M., & Kriston, L. (2008). St John's wort for major depression. *Cochrane.Database. Syst.Rev.*, CD000448.

Manu, P., Lane, T.J., & Matthews, D.A. (1993). Chronic fatigue and chronic fatigue syndrome: clinical epidemiology and aetiological classification. *Ciba Found.Symp.*, 173:23-31; discussion 31-42., 23-31.

Matsuda, Y., Matsui, T., Kataoka, K., Fukada, R., Fukuda, S., Kuratsune, H., Tajima, S., Yamaguti, K., Kato, Y.H., & Kiriike, N. (2009). A two-year follow-up study of chronic fatigue syndrome comorbid with psychiatric disorders. *Psychiatry Clin Neurosci.*, 63, 365-373.

Moskowitz, M. H., & Golden, M. (2013). *Neuroplastic Transformation.*

Nater, U.M., Jones, J.F., Lin, J.M., Maloney, E., Reeves, W.C., & Heim, C. (2010). Personality features and personality disorders in chronic fatigue syndrome: a population-based study. *Psychother. Psychosom.*, 79, 312-318.

Nater, U.M., Lin, J.M., Maloney, E.M., Jones, J.F., Tian, H., Boneva, R.S., Raison, C.L., Reeves, W.C., & Heim, C. (2009). Psychiatric comorbidity in persons with chronic fatigue syndrome identified from the Georgia population. *Psychosom.Med.*, 71, 557-565.

Pae, C.U., Luyten, P., Marks, D.M., Han, C., Park, S.H., Patkar, A.A., Masand, P.S., & Van, H.B. (2008). The relationship between fibromyalgia and major depressive disorder: a comprehensive review. *Curr. Med.Res.Opin.*, 24, 2359-2371.

Parlor, M. (2009). Profile and impact of 23 chronic conditions in the 2005 Canadian community health survey. *National ME/FM Action Network.*

Rahimi, R., Nikfar, S., & Abdollahi, M. (2009). Efficacy and tolerability of Hypericum perforatum in major depressive disorder in comparison with selective serotonin reuptake inhibitors: a meta-analysis. *Prog.Neuropsychopharmacol.Biol.Psychiatry*, 33, 118-127.

Raphael, K.G., Janal, M.N., Nayak, S., Schwartz, J.E., & Gallagher, R.M. (2006). Psychiatric comorbidities in a community sample of women with fibromyalgia. *Pain*, 124, 117-125.

Simon, G.E., Katon, W.J., & Sparks, P.J. (1990). Allergic to life: psychological factors in environmental illness. *Am. J Psychiatry*, 147, 901-906.

Sublette, M.E., Ellis, S.P., Geant, A.L., & Mann, J.J. (2011). Meta-analysis of the effects of eicosapentaenoic acid (EPA) in clinical trials in depression. *J Clin Psychiatry.*, 72, 1577-1584.

Swoboda, D.A. (2008). Negotiating the diagnostic uncertainty of contested illnesses: physician practices and paradigms. *Health (London)*, 12, 453-478.

Taylor, R.R. & Jason, L.A. (2001). Sexual abuse, physical abuse, chronic fatigue, and chronic fatigue syndrome: a community-based study. *J Nerv.Ment.Dis.*, 189, 709-715.

Thieme, K., Turk, D.C., & Flor, H. (2004). Comorbid depression and anxiety in fibromyalgia syndrome: relationship to somatic and psychosocial variables. *Psychosom.Med.*, 66, 837-844.

Torres-Harding, S.R., Jason, L.A., Cane, V., Carrico, A., & Taylor, R.R. (2002). Physicians' diagnoses of psychiatric disorders for people with chronic fatigue syndrome. *Int.J Psychiatry Med.*, 32, 109-124.

Vercoulen, J.H., Swanink, C.M., Zitman, F.G., Vreden, S.G., Hoofs, M.P., Fennis, J.F., Galama, J.M., van der Meer, J.W., & Bleijenberg, G. (1996). Randomised, double-blind, placebo-controlled study of fluoxetine in chronic fatigue syndrome. *Lancet*, 347, 858-861.

Wessely, S., Chalder, T., Hirsch, S., Wallace, P., & Wright, D. (1996). Psychological symptoms, somatic symptoms, and psychiatric disorder in chronic fatigue and chronic fatigue syndrome: a prospective study in the primary care setting. *American Journal of Psychiatry*, 153, 1050-1059.

Wessely, S., David, A., Butler, S., & Chalder, T. (1989). Management of chronic (post-viral) fatigue syndrome. *Journal of the Royal College of General Practitioners*, 39, 26-29.

Wessely, S., Nimnuan, C., & Sharpe, M. (1999). Functional somatic syndromes: one or many?. *Lancet*, 354, 936-939.

Wolfe, F., Hassett, A.L., Walitt, B., & Michaud, K. (2011). Mortality in fibromyalgia: a study of 8,186 patients over thirty-five years. *Arthritis Care Res.(Hoboken.)*, 63, 94-101.

Zheng, C. J., Van Drunen, S., & Egorova-Brumley, N. (2022). Neural correlates of co-occurring pain and depression: an activation-likelihood estimation (ALE) meta-analysis and systematic review. *Transl Psychiatry Psychiatry*, *12*(1), 196. https://doi.org/10.1038/s41398-022-01949-3

Session 9

Common Treatments

Every Day Is a New Day

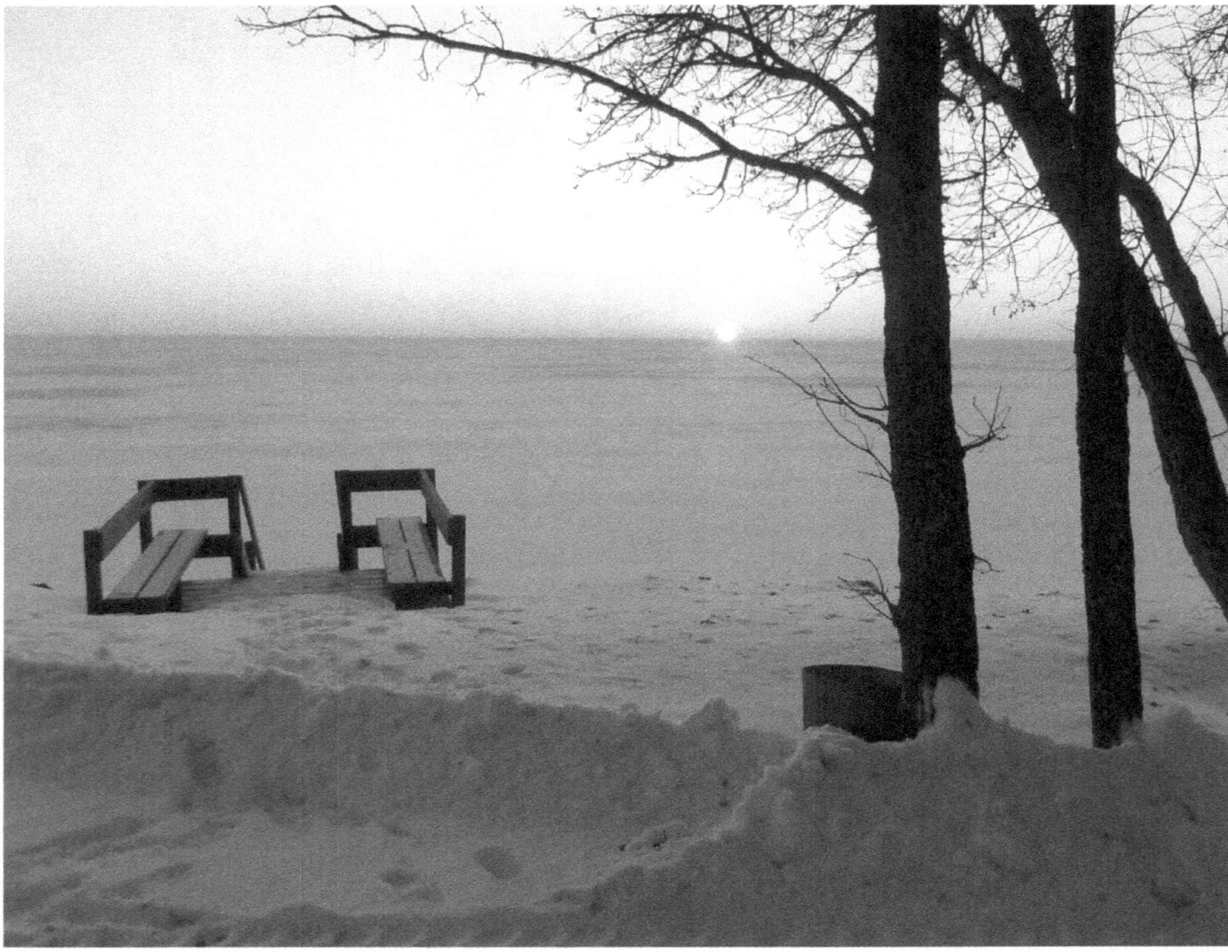

Graham Cox, Lake Winnipeg, Manitoba

Session 9

Common Treatment

Introduction

In this session, I mention specific products and tests that I find helpful for selected patients. The suggestions presented in this session are among those most commonly used by experts in the fields of ME/CFS, FM and MCS. However, because ME/CFS, FM and MCS are rarely taught in professional training programs (e.g., medical and nursing schools), your health care practitioner may be unfamiliar with these treatment strategies. I have included enough details and references here to enable you to discuss these ideas with your physician. However, be aware that some physicians may be reluctant to assist you with a strategy that they haven't learnt about before from a more authoritative source.

Most of these strategies have been fine-tuned over decades but lack the rigorous (usually double-blinded) research studies that modern physicians rely on to direct their practice. Be patient and look around for a health care professional who can help you decide whether any of these suggestions are suitable and safe for you.

- Any treatment with the power to heal also has the power to harm.
- Natural does not mean safe. Mercury and arsenic are naturally occurring substances that can kill.
- And just because a treatment has been scrutinized and studied does not mean that it is safe. Conventional medical care results in the deaths of tens of thousands of Canadians each year (Weingart et al., 2000).
- You need professional assistance to help you decide if any of the suggestions in this session may be of benefit to you.

Many patients yearn for a simple treatment program or algorithm to follow. There are algorithms for treatment in other fields of medicine, which I read with envy; how nice it would be if the path were this straightforward. Although there are some stepwise treatment protocols available in the field of ME/CFS and FM, such as those of Dr. Jacob Teitelbaum, Dr. Ritchie Shoemaker, and Dr. Paul Cheney, I have yet to find one path that works for everyone. And to be fair to these experienced, groundbreaking clinicians, in real life, they thoroughly assess each patient, and the paths of each can differ significantly.

Maybe in time, and with more research, it will all become clearer. But in the meantime, these suggestions must be considered individually. They are not part of a treatment protocol or program. Remember that if you try more than one new idea at a time, you will be unable to tell what made you better or worse. As with all the suggestions in this manual, please try/add/subtract one thing at a time. If something helps even a small amount, keep it in your management plan and look for something else to add to it. If an intervention doesn't help at all, either with how you feel or any laboratory parameters, then I would advise letting that one go and moving on. Even if you hear convincing testimonies about a treatment from other patients and practitioners, remember that we are all unique, and it may not work for you. Similarly, you may stumble upon something that works even when others don't benefit from it. We each have to find our own path to recovery.

Some points to keep in mind as you read this session:

- There are many good products and services available, including many that I have never heard of or tried. My selections are based on consensus in the field and my clinical experience.
- I have no financial interest in any medical-related company and benefit in no way from any recommendation in this manual or session.
- In deciding whether to try any new strategy, each patient must weigh the risks and benefits of the strategy with the risks and benefits of *care as usual*. Care as usual refers to what you would be doing if you didn't try a new intervention. In the fields of ME/CFS, FM and MCS care, as usual, generally means having an annual physical, having other conditions treated, and the ME/CFS, FM and MCS being entirely ignored. This is because most physicians are not aware of the strategies presented in this manual, nor the suggestions in this session.

  The research on care as usual for ME/CFS and FM highlights a lack of success. Follow-up studies show that there is little recovery over time for either ME/CFS or FM (Cairns & Hotopf, 2005; White & Harth, 2001). MCS has not been studied. It is hoped that symptomatic approaches, such as in this manual, will lead to improved outcomes compared with care as usual. However, until studies are done, we will not know for sure.

Try to read this session with an open mind, whether you are newly diagnosed or a veteran, whether you have already tried many remedies, or you are entirely new to this. If you have already tried a specific approach, there may be no need to revisit it. But remember that the body changes over time. For some patients, spending time on self-management, including medication or natural remedy trials, as appropriate, may increase health enough that some interventions that were previously unsuccessful become helpful when tried again. Your health care practitioner can help you decide whether this might be true for you.

Before you even consider the strategies in this session, remember that they are never used in isolation but rather in the context of many assumptions. **If any of the assumptions below are not true, then please don't proceed.**

Correct diagnosis: This requires a full medical assessment by a qualified health care professional, including a careful history (listening to your story), physical examination, and ruling out of other possible causes of your symptoms. Reread the diagnostic criteria listed in Session 1 carefully and review them with your physician. Make sure that you actually have ME/CFS, FM or MCS before proceeding.

Optimal self-management: Without self-management, i.e., having worked through the other eight sessions in this manual, these more specialized strategies may be of limited benefit. Self-management is necessary in all cases.

A collaborative relationship between you and your health care professional is critical. Health care professionals are advised to find a mentor to support them while learning new skills. There are many practitioners, both MDs and NDs, who use these treatments as part of their routine practice and may be willing to assist you.

Joan's Experience

When Joan read about these additional strategies, she took the manual to her family physician to ask for assistance so that she could try some that were relevant and safe for her. Joan heeded the advice in this manual and resisted her temptation to try some of the over-the-counter products without supervision.

Her family physician had not heard of any of these approaches and was not open to discussing them. Joan was very disappointed. She weighed the pros and cons of finding a new family physician; someone either more open-minded or more knowledgeable. However, Joan's family physician has been very proactive and helpful with respect to Joan's other medical problems. As a result, Joan decided not to switch, knowing that it could be very difficult to find a new doctor with the physician shortage in Canada. She then contacted her local FM support group and attended some meetings to meet members and ask for their recommendations as to other professionals who could help her.

A local Naturopathic Doctor (ND) was recommended by a couple of the support group members. Joan met with this ND to get information about how much she knew about FM and to discuss some of the recommendations in this manual. The ND said that she had treated many FM patients with success and was confident that she could help Joan. They met again for the practitioner to take a full history (the story of Joan's health problems). Immediately after the history taking, the ND told Joan that she had *adrenal fatigue* and *nutrient deficiencies*. Joan asked how the ND could know this without doing any testing. The ND said that she came to these conclusions based on Joan's symptom profile.

Joan, having read the manual, knew that although these things could be true for her, they also might not be, since the symptoms of many conditions overlap. She became wary. At this point, the practitioner became a bit defensive and angry. Joan felt uncomfortable and said she would think it over before embarking on the treatment plan. She left without purchasing any products.

After doing some more research, Joan found another ND in the area who also had experience with FM. With this practitioner, all the boxes of informed consent were checked off.

- This ND stated that he couldn't make any recommendations without further investigations into the most likely causes of Joan's symptoms.
- He added that in the past, he had, at times, been mistaken about the best way to proceed and felt more comfortable doing testing before recommending any treatment.
- He outlined how much the recommended investigations would cost, the probability that each one might lead to some change in treatment, and how much the possible treatments would cost.
- He also mentioned the risks and benefits of each potential treatment. Joan felt more comfortable with this approach, but was limited due to finances.
- She asked which of the tests the ND rated as the highest priority for her, and they reviewed the details of that test. She decided to go ahead with one test (unique for each person, so not being mentioned here) with the understanding that if the results were abnormal, Joan would try to treat the problem before moving on to any other testing or treatment.

Although the above is a typical story, I am revealing my bias here for testing rather than treating blindly. Not all practitioners agree with this approach. Some believe that they can discern physiology through history alone. I have seen many patients who had been told by a former practitioner that they had *candida* or *adrenal fatigue*, and subsequent appropriate testing was unable to detect these problems. Sometimes tests confirm these clinical diagnoses, and sometimes they don't.

Lest some feel at this point, I'm picking on NDs; incorrect assumptions can be made by any practitioner. I have made incorrect assumptions many times. Rather, I am focusing on NDs in this section since their training and expertise include the use of herbal and nutritional supplements. They are likely to be able to help when medication and conventional testing don't help. Many patients seek the professional advice of NDs and benefit from the care they receive. Like all other practitioners (including MDs), some NDs are excellent diagnosticians and some are sloppy.

Trust your intuition when seeking out any practitioner. And be particularly wary of any practitioner who makes a program sound too straightforward or easy, or who brags of too much success. The reality is that for ME/CFS, FM and MCS, the path is complicated and littered with false starts.

Test to Rule Out Treatable Contributors to Disease

In the fields of complex chronic diseases, most tests are done to rule things out rather than rule things in.

Recommended generally available tests include

- CBC + differential (the number of red and various white blood cells): To rule out blood disorders, especially anaemia.
- Electrolytes: To rule out dehydration, acidosis, or electrolyte imbalance.
- Liver function tests (e.g., GGT, ALT): To rule out liver damage of any cause.
- Thyroid-Stimulating Hormone (TSH): To rule out thyroid disorder.
- Anti-Nuclear Antibody (ANA), Rheumatoid Factor (RF): To rule out common rheumatological disorders.
- Iron indices: Serum iron, ferritin, total iron binding capacity and transferrin saturation: To rule out anemia, hemochromatosis and inflammation.
- Inflammatory markers, including Erythrocyte Sedimentation Rate (ESR), C-Reactive Protein (CRP) (discussed in Session 5), and fibrinogen: To rule out inflammation or infection.

Depending on your unique symptom profile, you may require additional tests to rule in or rule out specific conditions.

Accessing Tests Not Covered by Provincial Health Care

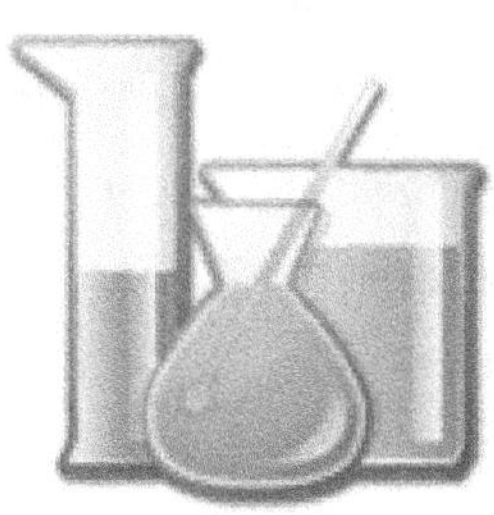

Throughout the manual, I refer to some laboratory tests that aren't available through provincial health care but that many patients find useful to help guide their health decisions. Most of these tests are available through private labs in the United States and Europe. These are approved labs that meet quality control and are operating legally. Like more routine tests, these alternative tests are only available through a health care professional (usually an MD or ND).

These tests often provide information about nutrition and function rather than about diagnosing a specific disease. Physicians who are experienced with these tests may be found through organizations such as the Institute of Functional Medicine or the Canadian Association of Naturopathic Doctors. The website of the provincial colleges and other professional associations often allows a search for keywords such as your illness or symptom.

Your family physician may be unfamiliar with tests outside the mainstream and skeptical that they are valid and useful. If you think that one of these fee-for-service tests might help you solve some puzzle about your health, you will have to find a practitioner who is able to guide you. Once you find a practitioner, be sure to inquire about the accuracy of the test and the relevance of the findings for your situation. Most importantly, ask if the test result changes your management plan.

Remember that no test is 100% accurate and that the test result may be *negative* (i.e., may not explain why you are ill). Therefore, ask yourself how you will feel if the test result is negative or if it doesn't help you with your health decisions. Will you still feel it was worth the money spent? Never spend money on testing that you need for other things, such as rent and food.

After discussing a test with your practitioner, and if you decide to go ahead, s/he will give you a test kit. A kit contains the laboratory requisition (which needs to be signed by your practitioner), the correct containers to collect blood, urine, saliva or stool (depending on the test), information about shipping, and shipping envelopes. Make sure to read all the instructions carefully to know where the sample is being shipped to and how soon it needs to get there.

Most large American labs have separate price lists for Canadian customers. With many labs, you will get a slightly cheaper price if you pay the practitioner up front and the practitioner pays the lab when you actually do the test. This is because there is less work involved for the lab to ensure payment from a health care professional who has registered with the lab. Many practitioners charge an added fee to cover the time it takes them to read and interpret your test results. Sometimes research or consultation is required of the practitioner. Remember, if the test is offered by a US lab, the fee will generally be in US Dollars. As the exchange rate varies, this can significantly affect the price.

Outside the Canadian publicly funded system, there are many tests which, although not diagnostic, can identify contributors to ill health. These contributors can be triggers of ME/CFS, FM or MCS or be factors that prevent recovery. There are hundreds of tests available through private laboratories. Many of these tests are helpful in individual cases. None are useful in every case as there is no single cause for these conditions. See Session 1 for details about how to access tests not offered through the Canadian public health care system and Session 5 for tests related to nutrition and gut health.

Here are a few of the most clinically useful and cost-efficient tests that I use in my practice. All are done at Clinical Laboratory Improvement Amendments (known as CLIA) certified (i.e., respected, not fly-by-night) labs in the US. Most of these labs offer consultation by phone to ordering physicians to help them interpret tests with which they may not be familiar.

Chelation Challenged 24-hour Urine for Heavy Metals

Rationale: Heavy metals such as lead, mercury, cadmium, and others have an adverse impact on health. Identifying and decreasing the body burden of heavy metals may lead to improved health. There continues to be much debate about whether chelation (the treatment of taking a drug that will bind to and facilitate the excretion of heavy metals) will help any, some, or most people who have elevated body burdens. My opinion is that while it may not help everyone, it is better not to have these toxins in the body. So, for those who can afford to do so and are able to tolerate the treatment, I recommend testing for heavy metals.

Procedure: A chelation-challenged urine collection is considered the gold standard test for heavy metal body burden. A chelation challenge may be done by IV 2, 3-Dimercapto-1-propanesulfonic acid (DMPS), or oral Dimercaptosuccinic acid (DMSA). IV Chelation should only be done by practitioners who have American College for Advancement in Medicine (ACAM) or similar certification showing competence in this skill. There are many such practitioners, both MDs and NDs, in Calgary and across the country. Many labs offer heavy metal testing of various body fluids and tissues. I use the US lab, Doctor's Data, for heavy metal testing.

Benefits: Identification of a potential determinant of ill health that can be remedied.

Risks: Adverse reaction to the chelating chemicals—this can be unpleasant but rarely serious. Adverse reactions can be reactions to the chelating chemicals themselves or due to the mobilization of heavy metals.

Complete Biochemistry Panel

Rationale: It is possible to test for many critical nutritional metabolites, including fatty acids, amino acids, organic acids, oxidative markers, and heavy metals. These tests also give information on the functioning of many important reactions in the body, such as the citric acid (energy) cycle and the function of many minerals and vitamins. Note that few panels measure mineral and vitamin levels directly. Vitamin levels in the body, especially water-soluble ones, change all the time and testing them directly is not considered valid or useful.

Instead, the function of essential elements can be measured indirectly through the biochemistry panel. Through this testing, one can learn if the food one is eating is actually getting to where it needs to go and doing the job it needs to do. Some inborn (genetic) metabolic problems or pathways blocked by toxins can also be identified. Optimal health and recovery from illness require that all metabolic pathways are functioning as well as possible. A biochemistry panel measures some of the more common and critical pathways and metabolites to assess function.

Procedure: For this panel, I recommend the US lab Genova's *Ion Panel*.

Benefits: Identification of nutritional and metabolic problems that are treatable with nutritional supplementation. With this information, patients may be able to save money on supplements that are found to be unnecessary and instead spend their resources on the most significant issues that are identified.

Risks: The test may fail to show any abnormalities. Or it may identify problems that are hard to fix. This can be stressful.

Testing for Lyme Disease

Rationale: The symptoms of chronic Lyme Disease are very similar to those of ME/CFS and FM. Lyme Disease is an infectious disease caused by the Borrelia burgdorferi bacteria, spread by Ixodes deer ticks (both Ixodes scapularis and Ixodes pacificus). Although the nature of acute Lyme Disease is not contentious, the presence of chronic Lyme Disease is.

Many, including infectious disease specialists, believe that chronic Lyme Disease doesn't exist, exists but not in Canada, or exists but is easily treatable. Members of the organization ILADS (International Lyme and Associated Diseases Society) believe that chronic Lyme disease is a serious disorder consisting of neurological and physical symptoms, which is found all over the world and is often resistant to antibiotic treatments.

Research shows that deer ticks infected with Borrelia burgdorferi, the causative agent for Lyme disease, exist in every province in Canada (Sperling & Sperling, 2009). The Public Health Agency of Canada has an information sheet with information about tick identification at http://www.phac-aspc.gc.ca/id-mi/tickinfo-eng.php.

ELISA antibody tests, such as the one currently used by the Canadian health care system, have a sensitivity of 5% - 60% (Ang et al., 2011; Wojciechowska-Koszko et al., 2011; Ogden et al., 2011). This means 40% or more of patients who have contracted Lyme disease will have a false negative result.

If a patient has engaged in outdoor activities in Borrelia endemic areas (they are present in every province, but the risk is highest in the warmer climates), a review of the symptoms of Lyme disease should be undertaken, and testing considered. The International Lyme and Associated Diseases Society (ILADS) website http://www.ilads.org/ has information on symptomatology of Lyme Disease, as well as the unique symptoms of the other pathogens that are transmitted with Borrelia by deer ticks.

Common co-infections of Lyme Disease include Babesia, Ehrlichia, and Bartonella. The ILADS website also has links to sites outlining the position of the Infectious Disease Society of America (IDSA), which espouses opposing views on chronic Lyme disease to those expressed by the ILADS.

Procedure: Given the many false negatives from the testing currently available from the public system in Canada, I recommend the Western Blot test as offered at IGenex lab in the US, www.igenex.com (or other labs). This test is also imperfect, but it has a much better sensitivity than the ELISA.

Risks: If a positive result occurs, it may be very hard to find a physician in Canada willing and able to treat adequately. And if you are especially unlucky, you may find yourself in the middle of the heated political debate between physicians who believe that chronic Lyme Disease exists and those who don't.

Benefits: If you can afford treatment in BC, where NDs now have the ability and training to prescribe for Lyme Disease, or to go to the US for assessment and treatment with a Lyme-literate physician, significantly improved health is possible.

General Nutritional Supplementation

Many patients with ME/CFS, FM and MCS feel that they are nutritionally depleted or that they are not eating well enough to recover their health. While nothing beats real food, for various reasons, a healthy diet is not possible for all patients. Some patients report feeling better when they take a general nutritional supplement. I frequently recommend the following products.

Fatigued to Fantastic Energy Revitalization System®

This nutrient powder is one part of Dr. Teitelbaum's entire treatment protocol/program. Dr. Jacob Teitelbaum is a pioneer in the field of fibromyalgia. He is an internist and FM survivor who has developed the *Fatigued to Fantastic* treatment program based on empirical experience rather than an underlying etiological hypothesis. His double-blind placebo-controlled treatment trial of his entire program (i.e., not just the powder) (Teitelbaum et al., 2000) shows significantly better results than any other published trial in either CFS or FM. 29/32 patients with FM on active treatment improved versus only 12/32 patients on a placebo program.

Dr. Teitelbaum's entire treatment protocol is based on supplementing or treating all symptoms and the underlying health problems they may represent. For many patients, this results in a complex mix of nutritional supplements and medications. Dr. Teitelbaum has been criticized by physicians in the field for using the "kitchen sink" approach (i.e., using too many things at once). Dr. T. argues back, explaining that if one has a car that isn't working, one must ensure every part of the car is repaired before it will run smoothly. He believes the same is true of the human body.

The nutrient powder designed by Dr. Teitelbaum is well-tolerated and reported to be effective by many patients. The powder contains whey protein (problematic for people with a milk allergy), minerals, vitamins, and several additional ingredients thought to be helpful for people with FM. These include malate (helps with energy), several free-form amino acids, grape seed extract (helps with oxidative stress), and choline (helps build healthy fat).

For more information, go to Dr. Teitelbaum's website: www.endfatigue.com/. You will find information about his treatment protocol and a link to a store that sells products he recommends.

Dose: The powder is taken at a dose of one scoop per day, mixed with water or juice. It is also available in a pre-measured, single-dose packet format.

Benefits: Many people report an overall improved sense of well-being, some people note no difference, and some unlucky ones have an adverse reaction.

Risks: As with any multi-ingredient product, patients with sensitivities may be unable to tolerate any number of ingredients, including the whey powder. Review the list of ingredients carefully before deciding whether this product is right for you.

Metagenics Ultraclear® and Sustain®

Two other "medical food" products, which are of benefit to many patients, are Ultraclear and Sustain, two of a large medical food line produced by Metagenics. A medical food includes as many of the essential nutrients as possible to combine into one product. Ultraclear® is one of Metagenics' oldest products and was formulated to assist with cognitive function in patients with ME/CFS. Sustain® is formulated to improve *leaky gut*.

Patients who are at risk of or have developed metabolic syndrome (discussed in Session 5) may also benefit from several newer formulations of these products (e.g., Ultraclear Plus®), which include products that help balance sugar and fat metabolism. However, some patients with ME/CFS, FM and MCS don't tolerate the additional ingredients. For this reason, I stick with these two tried and true products, which are generally well tolerated. Both Ultraclear® and Sustain® use a rice protein base to which the other supplements are added.

Dose: The powder is taken at a dose of two scoops per day, mixed with water or juice.

Available: These supplements are widely available from selected compounding pharmacies and practitioners such as Naturopathic Doctors and Chiropractors.

Benefits: Many people report an overall improved sense of well-being as well as improved gastrointestinal function with Sustain®.

Risks: As with any multi-ingredient product, patients with sensitivities may be unable to tolerate any number of ingredients, including the rice protein. Review the list of ingredients carefully before deciding whether this product is right for you.

High Dose B12

High-dose vitamin B12 has been used for ME/CFS since the 1950s, though it is only recently that we have a putative hypothesis about why it helps. B12 is a nitric oxide scavenger. Nitric oxide (NO) augments oxidative pathways (Pall, 2001). Nitric oxide pathways are known to be augmented in ME/CFS, and oxidative damage is increased in both ME/CFS and FM (Khan et al., 2003; Richards et al., 2007).

Multiple chemical sensitivity has not been studied in this way, but Dr. Martin Pall hypothesizes that MCS may be maintained by a similar process. High-dose B12 is also used in other chronic conditions that affect the central nervous system.

Based on imaging studies, we know that ME/CFS, FM and MCS all affect the central nervous system. In ME/CFS and MCS, there is decreased and spotty brain blood flow on SPECT scans (Schwartz et al., 1994; Orriols et al., 2009). In both ME/CFS and FM, there is diminished gray matter volume on specialized MRI tests (de Lange et al., 2005; Lutz et al., 2008). This is a treatment for which we have no randomized trial evidence, only the clinical experience of dozens of physicians over the past 60 years to guide us.

Protocol: There are different protocols. Some clinicians prefer to use hydroxy B12, and some prefer methyl B12. Both penetrate the CNS. CNS penetration is thought to be critical for effectiveness. The Pall protocol (see treatment 9 in this session) recommends sublingual hydroxy B12, but all others in the field recommend injection or nebulized (turning liquid into a mist which is then inhaled) administration. In my practice, the sublingual form has not proved to be effective. Injection is recommended by virtually all ME/CFS practitioners, whereas nebulized B12 is recommended in some MCS protocols. I have not been able to ascertain which is better in my practice.

NOTE: This protocol does not use cyanocobalamin (Cyano B12). Cyano B12 is the commonly used form of B12 given by injection to elderly patients with low B12 levels. Cyano B12 should not be used in high doses. Cyano B12 does not increase energy and cognitive function unless there is a B12 deficiency. There is no evidence that patients with ME/CFS, FM or MCS have a B12 deficiency, and the high-dose protocol recommended here is not being used with the purpose of fixing a deficiency. I can't highlight this point clearly enough because even with this emphasis, many people get confused.

Using B12 at high (pharmacological) doses has the objective of decreasing nitric oxide synthesis and oxidation in the brain. Methyl and hydroxy B12 can improve symptoms of ME/CFS, FM and MCS regardless of serum B12 levels (which will be high after a couple of doses).

Dose: 10mg/ml methyl or hydroxy B12 X 1ml by IM, SC injection or nebulizer 2-3 times weekly. Most patients can be taught to safely administer their own injections. Many MCS protocols combine the B12 with reduced glutathione, 1mL of 100mg/mL at each dose.

Available: Injectable B12 is available by prescription only. You must find a qualified MD or ND to prescribe this for you.

Benefits: Patients report improved cognitive function and stamina. B12 should be used for a month or so before assessing its effectiveness. However, some patients report benefit after the first injection.

Risks: A review of the world literature (admittedly small and inadequate) turns up no reports of adverse effects. In my practice and from discussions with colleagues who use this treatment routinely, the only side effects noted are occasional bruising or soreness at the injection site and the ever-present risk of infection if sterile technique is not followed. There is one case in the literature of a non-fatal allergy developing over time. It is best to request preservative-free injectables to decrease the risk of allergy. This means, however, that the product will have a shorter *fridge life*. B12 must be kept refrigerated. Patients should be screened for bleeding disorders (e.g., INR, platelet count), and those with low or borderline counts should be advised to use a nebulizer instead of injections.

Increasing Blood Volume

If you do not have any of the symptoms mentioned in the autonomic nervous system section of Session 3, and especially if your BP is normal or high, the following treatment is **not** indicated.

I introduced information about heart rate variability in Session 3. Using heart rate variability as a measure, it has been repeatedly shown that there is significant autonomic dysfunction in both ME/CFS and FM (Hurwitz, 2002; Cohen et al., 2001). In ME/CFS, this abnormality is thought to be, at least in part, due to decreased red blood cell (RBC) mass and blood volume (Streeten & Bell, 1998).

Clinically, I have observed urgent urination followed by dizziness and light-headedness, which are frequently reported in MCS after an exposure. This fluid loss may lead to similar problems with low blood volume.

Since it is not currently possible to measure blood volume or RBC mass through the Canadian public health care system, one must use blood pressure, heart rate, heart rate variability, and clinical symptoms as an indicator. I recommend the NASA lean test described in Session 3 to see if you may have low blood volume or pressure.

Remember that even in 2025, many MDs don't consider low blood pressure to be a problem. Finding someone to work with you may be a challenge. However, as with all the other recommendations in this session, you need professional assistance. You should not undertake changing your blood volume without it.

Protocol: Increasing blood volume with salt/electrolyte and fluid loading is the safest and least expensive method. Whether using sea salt or an electrolyte mix, use your salt-and-water supplement as a "drug." This means taking a measured amount at regular intervals so that the appropriate dose can be fine-tuned to BP, HR, and symptoms. Increasing the resting BP to the normal range of 120/80 and decreasing the resting HR to below 90 bpm can result in feeling better.

A typical dose of sea salt is 1/4 - 1/2 tsp up to four times daily, or an electrolyte mix 1/8 -1/4 tsp up to three times daily. If you are chemically sensitive or have MCAS, try to find a powdered mix without colors or flavors.

Some people are having success with World Health Organization oral rehydration solutions. These are a mixture of saltwater and glucose. This recipe is used for people who are dehydrated from diarrhea from things like cholera. The glucose assists the sodium in entering the blood. There are ready-made products like Trioral®, Ceralyte 90®, and Liquid IV® that meet the WHO guidelines for oral rehydration. Or you can learn how to make the solution yourself on YouTube.

Benefits: Increased blood volume in a person with previously low blood volume may lead to increases in energy and cognitive function. As resting heart rate decreases, exercise capacity may improve.

Risks: Patients must monitor BP regularly to ensure they don't overshoot. Short-term increases in BP above the normal range (120/80) pose little risk and can be quickly corrected by decreasing the dose of electrolyte or salt.

Free Form Amino Acids

Patients with ME/CFS, FM and MCS seem to require a higher and more consistent protein intake than healthy people. Whereas most health recommendations are to eat less meat, patients with ME/CFS, FM and MCS rarely thrive on a vegetarian diet. We now know that this is due to problems with energy metabolism that result in protein being burned for energy in preference to carbohydrates (Fluge et al., 2016).

Amino acids are the molecules from which protein is constructed. There are approximately 21 structural amino acids. They have names like glycine, glutamine, cysteine, proline, and valine. Some amino acids must be obtained from the diet. These are called the *essential amino acids*. Essential refers to any nutrient that must be obtained from the diet because the body cannot make it from other nutrients. The other amino acids can be transformed from the essentials.

Note that amino acids are not the same as organic acids, the testing of which has been discussed in Session 2, in the section on L-tryptophan (itself an amino acid), and in Session 5, in the section on dysbiosis.

Many private labs in the US offer tests for amino acid levels in the body. I prefer a 24-hour urine profile over the serum test. If the levels are low for most or all amino acids, I look for evidence of insufficient protein intake, poor digestion or poor absorption. The same test measures excretion of muscle metabolic products such as 1-methylhistidine and 3-methylhistidine. When high, these measures suggest that the increased protein needs may be due to muscle degradation.

> *Test*: 24-hour urine for amino acids.
>
> *Available*: Doctor's Data Laboratory and others in the US.
>
> *Test*: The ION biochemical panel mentioned in Treatment 1 of this session also includes a measure of amino acids.
>
> *Protocol*: Ensure adequate protein intake by taking regular servings of animal-sourced (i.e., complete) protein each day. Chew food thoroughly. If needed, use digestive enzymes to ensure optimal digestion. Digestive enzymes are discussed in Session 5.
>
> For some reason, my patients report that the use of commercial protein powder seems less effective than the use of free-form (already digested) amino acids. However, protein powder, especially undenatured whey protein, is recommended by some in the field. Undenatured whey protein is purified at a lower temperature than many protein powders. This protects some of the

valuable protein components, such as lactoferrin. Undenatured whey powder may not be tolerated by people with milk allergies.

Free-form amino acids should be tolerated by the vast majority of patients since they do not retain traces of the proteins from which they were derived and are naturally found in every cell of our bodies.

Dose: 1 tsp free-form amino powder with water or juice in the morning before eating.

Benefits: May increase energy and cognitive function.

Risks: Amino acids are powerful molecules. Some, such as glycine and aspartate, are neurotransmitters. Only use amino acids under the supervision of a health care professional. Some patients find the taste objectionable due to the sulphur-containing amino acids. Patients with sulphur or sulphate allergies should use it with caution. One should use a mixed and balanced amino acid product since the use of large amounts of single amino acids prevents absorption by others through competition for transporters.

Magnesium

Magnesium is a muscle relaxant. Since so many patients with FM have increased muscle tension (Donaldson et al., 2002b; Donaldson et al., 2002a), there are many clinicians who, based on symptom profile, believe that patients with FM are depleted in magnesium. Although a few small studies support this belief, it has not been widely validated (Keenoy et al., 2000).

Part of the problem is the difficulty in measuring intracellular mineral levels accurately. A measure of magnesium in red blood cells is a way to measure how much is in cells in general. In Canada, RBC magnesium is difficult to access.

NOTE: The regular serum (extracellular) magnesium test is not of value for evaluating intracellular stores.

Protocol: Bowel tolerance to oral magnesium varies widely. Effective doses for muscle relaxation varied from about 250 mg up to three times per day, up to 2 - 3 g/day. Mg can also be taken by injection. The usual recommended dose is 50% Mg Sulphate 0.2 – 0.5 mg three times weekly to three times daily. The injections can be given either subcutaneously or intramuscularly. Most patients can be taught to safely administer their own injections. The injections can be discontinued when the symptoms are alleviated, often after about 3 months.

Benefits: Magnesium may decrease muscle pain, tension, and cramping, especially in patients with FM. Improved sleep and improved bowel function, if constipated, are positive side effects.

Risks: Diarrhea occurs if oral magnesium is dosed beyond bowel tolerance. In people with loose stools already, oral magnesium may not be tolerated. Injections can cause flushing and sweating. High-dose IV treatment (not advocated here) for intractable seizures can cause muscle relaxation and respiratory depression.

Testing for and Eliminating Toxic Mould

In his book *Desperation Medicine* (Shoemaker, 2001), Dr. Ritchie Shoemaker explains how he has successfully treated patients with multiple complex chronic conditions by detoxifying from mold and mycotoxins. He hypothesizes that in the people he has successfully treated, there was a previously unknown cause: biotoxins. Biotoxins are small molecules produced by a number of infective agents, including ciguatera dinoflagellates living in fish, Borrelia, the infection causing Lyme disease, and Stachybotrys, and other moulds which grow in water-damaged buildings. Shoemaker believes that it is these biotoxins, often unrecognized, that cause many of the symptoms of the above health conditions.

Shoemaker lists the following as typical symptoms of biotoxin exposure:

- Severe headaches worsen with exposure to light, especially fluorescents.
- Muscle aches all over and a long recovery time from exercise.
- Poor memory, poor concentration, and brain fog.
- Blurred vision.
- Numbness of extremities.
- Severe fatigue.
- Bowel spasms.

I am only discussing one of these biotoxins here: those produced by mold. The health hazards of indoor, toxic mold must be differentiated from the mostly benign effects of outdoor, ambient moulds. There is mold almost everywhere, all the time. Antarctica may be a possible exception. We breathe mold spores and mold metabolites all the time, and most people are not adversely affected. An exception is people with mold allergies who get hay fever and asthma symptoms at the times of year when outdoor moulds grow.

Mold that grows in the walls and ceilings of water-damaged buildings is often toxic. People can become allergic to this mould as well as suffer from the effects of the toxic substances the mould makes and releases into the air (Straus, 2009). The evidence suggests that patients living in mouldy indoor environments will not be able to recover their health until the leaks are repaired and the mouldy area is remediated.

Procedure: If you can see the mold and have confidence that you know the source of the problem, you should not need to get the air in your house tested. Skip to assessing what to do about the mold problem. If you are not sure if you have a mold problem, there are a number of different techniques that can be used to check for mold. I mention only two here. The traditional method of mould testing is to hire an air quality inspector to come to the house and search for signs of moisture.

Agar plates are left in suspected areas for a few days. The plates are then taken to a lab to see if any toxin-producing mold species are growing. The benefits of this approach are that one has a quantitative measure of how much mold is present, along with which species are growing and the area of the dwelling in which the mold is located. The downside is that sometimes mold, which grew happily in the damp wall space, doesn't grow so well on the agar plate, and measurements can be misleading.

An alternative strategy is called the Environmental Relative Moldiness Index (ERMI). This test may be available through air quality inspectors. The kit includes an attachment that fits on the end of your vacuum. You are instructed to vacuum the air, carpet, etc., of the two rooms in which you spend the most time. You then return the air/dust sample to the lab, and the lab measures the dust for the DNA of various mould species, both common ambient outdoor species and toxic indoor species. This gives a very accurate assessment of how many spores of both indoor and outdoor moulds are inside your residence. Health problems only occur when indoor species far outnumber outdoor ones. The downside to this method is that if your house dust contains toxic mould species, you will still need assistance to determine exactly where the mould is growing so that you can get it remediated.

If you discover that you have moisture damage and toxic mould growth where you live, it must be fixed for your health to improve. If you are renting a dwelling and the landlord is unwilling to take the problem seriously, you may need to move. If you own the dwelling, then it is your responsibility to fix the problem. If it is a small problem, you may be able to do the remediation yourself. References abound on the internet about how to go about it, but be cautious and wear a mask. The Canada Mortgage and Housing Corporation provides useful information on identifying and remediating mould from water damage. https://assets.cmhc-schl.gc.ca/sf/project/cmhc/pdfs/content/en/mould-information-for-occupants.pdf?rev=e0221968-4b08-4320-8d17-b98470c3c264

Remediating mold can be costly. Sometimes the cost is covered by insurance, but often not. Make sure you find a company experienced with safe mould remediation so that disturbing the mold doesn't make you worse. Some buildings are so badly affected (e.g., former grow operations) that remediation is not possible. These expensive decisions can be very emotionally difficult. Consider what your health is worth to you. Can you afford not to act?

Available: For an ERMI (or the cheaper HERTSMI) test kit, go to www.mycometrics.com. Finding a qualified indoor air quality inspector can be tricky; not all are adequately trained. It is best to use someone who has been recommended by someone you trust, such as your physician.

You can get more information about indoor air quality at the Canadian Council of Occupational Health and Safety website: http://www.ccohs.ca/. The Environmental Health Association of Ontario website http://ehaontario.ca/ provides information (or links to it) about mould remediation. As well, it lists links to similar non-profit associations in other provinces (Nova Scotia, Quebec and Alberta). Contacts at these organizations may be able to recommend qualified inspectors.

Sauna + Cholestyramine

Sauna and cholestyramine have both already been covered individually in Session 6. This section provides a bit more background. While the technique of avoidance decreases the immediate symptoms of MCS due to decreased exposures, it may not lead to decreased sensitivity to unavoidable exposures.

At first, avoidance may cause just the opposite, increased sensitivity to unavoidable exposures. This phenomenon is called *unmasking*. It is thought that when people are frequently or continually exposed to toxins, they become masked—maybe the body is too exhausted to keep signalling danger when no action is taken, and it learns to ignore signals. Then, as the body learns again to react to signals, symptoms can unexpectedly increase. The masking hypothesis is purely speculative. However, it is frequently noted that when exposure decreases, the symptoms to future exposures can worsen before they improve. This tends to make people worry that they are getting worse when, in fact, they are taking the right steps. To improve long-term health, it is believed that one must lower the total load of toxins in the body.

Toxins can be excreted through urine, stool, bile, and sweat. Many of the most toxic chemicals are fat-soluble and are stored in fat. The body has few ways of excreting toxins stored in fat. It has been found that sweating is one of the few ways to increase excretion through the skin of fat-soluble chemicals (Rea, 1997). Sauna is used in Japan as a treatment for severe heart disease, suggesting that it is very safe from a cardiovascular perspective (Kihara et al., 2002). Sauna has been shown to increase excretion of some toxins that are not excreted in urine or stool (Genuis et al., 2011).

Other toxins can be excreted in bile, and the use of the bile sequestrant cholestyramine increases excretion through the stool by preventing reabsorption (Genuis et al., 2011; Genuis et al., 2010; Shoemaker & House, 2006). Dr. Ritchie Shoemaker believes that cholestyramine can help decrease the burden of toxins from many biological sources, including mould, Borrelia bacteria, and Pfiesteria (toxic algae).

> *Protocol*: You should begin sauna therapy at a relatively low temperature (approximately 50 degrees C) and gradually increase until you are sweating profusely. Sweating should come on slowly over 20–30 minutes and then continue for another 20 minutes as tolerated. Certain supplements, such as the B and C vitamins, taken before a sauna are thought to help the body deal with the oxidative stress of mobilized toxins.
>
> As mentioned in Session 6, cholestyramine is used to pull toxins from the gastrointestinal tract into the stool so that they will not be reabsorbed. The recommended dose of cholestyramine is 4g in water or juice taken up to four times daily, including right after a sauna. Cholestyramine must be taken two or more hours after food or supplements and 30 minutes before food. This makes it difficult to take all four doses in a day. I recommend using cholestyramine in whatever number of doses you can fit into your management plan rather than dismissing it as too hard.
>
> *Benefits*: A person should feel excellent after each sauna. Over time, the excretion of toxins may lead to overall improved health.
>
> *Risks*: Intense sweating can lead to dehydration. Always drink at least 1L of water with each sauna. BP and HR should be monitored to ensure strain on the body is not excessive. Too much toxic mobilization can occur, making a person feel worse instead of better after a sauna. If this occurs, decrease the temperature and duration and work up slowly until you are able to tolerate higher temperatures and increased sweating.

You have reached the end of the sessions. If you want guidance to put all of this information into action, consider the self-study online course I developed based on this manual. It is called *Pathways to Improvement* and consists of (you guessed it) 9 modules. Each module provides video lessons and focuses on the most helpful strategies I have learned over the past 25 years. https://www.eleanorsteinmd.ca/pathways

But before you wrap up, I have included a special bonus chapter to let you know about some of the exciting new information I have learned since the manual was first published, information that is transforming how I live my life and what I recommend to others.

Session 9 References

Akkus, S., Naziroglu, M., Eris, S., Yalman, K., Yilmaz, N., & Yener, M. (2009). Levels of lipid peroxidation, nitric oxide, and antioxidant vitamins in plasma of patients with fibromyalgia. *Cell Biochem.Funct.*

Ang, C.W., Notermans, D.W., Hommes, M., Simoons-Smit, A.M., & Herremans, T. (2011). Large differences between test strategies for the detection of anti-Borrelia antibodies are revealed by comparing eight ELISAs and five immunoblots. *Eur.J Clin Microbiol.Infect.Dis.*, 30, 1027-1032.

Bralley, J. & Lord, R. (1994). Treatment of Chronic Fatigue Syndrome with specific amino acid supplementation. *Journal of Applied Nutrition*, 46, 74-79.

Cairns, R. & Hotopf, M. (2005). A systematic review describing the prognosis of chronic fatigue syndrome. *Occup.Med (Lond)*, 55, 20-31.

Cohen, H., Neumann, L., Kotler, M., & Buskila, D. (2001). Autonomic nervous system derangement in fibromyalgia syndrome and related disorders. *Isr.Med.Assoc.J*, 3, 755-760.

de Lange, F.P., Kalkman, J.S., Bleijenberg, G., Hagoort, P., van der Meer, J.W., & Toni, I. (2005). Gray matter volume reduction in the chronic fatigue syndrome. *Neuroimage.*, 26, 777-781.

Donaldson, C.C., MacInnis, A.L., Snelling, L.S., Sella, G.E., & Mueller, H.H. (2002a). Characteristics of diffuse muscular coactivation (DMC) in persons with fibromyalgia -- part 2. (Abstract). *NeuroRehabilitation.*, 17, 41-48.

Donaldson, C.C., Snelling, L.S., MacInnis, A.L., Sella, G.E., & Mueller, H.H. (2002b). Diffuse muscular coactivation (DMC) as a potential source of pain in fibromyalgia -- part 1. (Abstract). *NeuroRehabilitation.*, 17, 33-39.

Fluge, Ø., Mella, O., Bruland, O., Risa, K., Dyrstad, S. E., Alme, K., . . . Fosså, A. (2016). Metabolic profiling indicates impaired pyruvate dehydrogenase function in myalgic encephalopathy/chronic fatigue syndrome. *JCI insight, 1*(21). doi:https://dx.doi.org/10.1172/jci.insight.89376

Genuis, S.J., Birkholz, D., Ralitsch, M., & Thibault, N. (2010). Human detoxification of perfluorinated compounds. *Public Health*, 124, 367-375.

Genuis, S.J., Birkholz, D., Rodushkin, I., & Beesoon, S. (2011). Blood, urine, and sweat (BUS) study: monitoring and elimination of bioaccumulated toxic elements. *Arch.Environ.Contam Toxicol.*, 61, 344-357.

Hurwitz, B. (2002). RBC mass, autonomic nervous system integrity and syncope susceptibility in chronic fatigue syndrome. National Institute of Allergy and Infectious Diseases.

Keenoy, B., Moorkens, G., Vertommen, J., Noe, M., Neve, J., & De, L. (2000). Magnesium status and parameters of the oxidant-antioxidant balance in patients with chronic fatigue: effects of supplementation with magnesium. *J.Am.Coll.Nutr.*, 19, 374-382.

Kennedy, G., Spence, V.A., McLaren, M., Hill, A., Underwood, C., & Belch, J.J. (2005). Oxidative stress levels are raised in chronic fatigue syndrome and are associated with clinical symptoms. *Free Radic.Biol.Med.*, 39, 584-589.

Khan, F., Spence, V., Kennedy, G., & Belch, J.J. (2003). Prolonged acetylcholine-induced vasodilatation in the peripheral microcirculation of patients with chronic fatigue syndrome. *Clin Physiol Funct. Imaging*, 23, 282-285.

Kihara, T., Biro, S., Imamura, M., Yoshifuku, S., Takasaki, K., Ikeda, Y., Otuji, Y., Minagoe, S., Toyama, Y., & Tei, C. (2002). Repeated sauna treatment improves vascular endothelial and cardiac function in patients with chronic heart failure. *J.Am.Coll.Cardiol.*, 39, 754-759.

Lutz, J., Jager, L., de, Q.D., Krauseneck, T., Padberg, F., Wichnalek, M., Beyer, A., Stahl, R., Zirngibl, B., Morhard, D., Reiser, M., & Schelling, G. (2008). White and gray matter abnormalities in the brain of patients with fibromyalgia: a diffusion-tensor and volumetric imaging study. *Arthritis Rheum.*, 58, 3960-3969.

Niblett, S.H., King, K.E., Dunstan, R.H., Clifton-Bligh, P., Hoskin, L.A., Roberts, T.K., Fulcher, G.R., McGregor, N.R., Dunsmore, J.C., Butt, H.L., Klineberg, I., & Rothkirch, T.B. (2007). Hematologic and urinary excretion anomalies in patients with chronic fatigue syndrome. *Exp.Biol.Med.(Maywood.)*, 232, 1041-1049.

Ogden, N.H., Margos, G., Aanensen, D.M., Drebot, M.A., Feil, E.J., Hanincova, K., Schwartz, I., Tyler, S., & Lindsay, L.R. (2011). Investigation of genotypes of Borrelia burgdorferi in Ixodes scapularis ticks collected during surveillance in Canada. *Appl.Environ.Microbiol.*, 77, 3244-3254.

Orriols, R., Costa, R., Cuberas, G., Jacas, C., Castell, J., & Sunyer, J. (2009). Brain dysfunction in multiple chemical sensitivity. *J.Neurol.Sci.*, 287, 72-78.

Pall, M.L. (2001). Cobalamin used in chronic fatigue syndrome therapy is a nitric oxide scavenger. *Journal of the Chronic Fatigue Syndrome*, 8, 39-44.

Pall, M.L. (2002). NMDA sensitization and stimulation by peroxynitrite, nitric oxide, and organic solvents as the mechanism of chemical sensitivity in multiple chemical sensitivity. *FASEB J*, 16, 1407-1417.

Rea, W. (1997) *Chemical Sensitivity,* CRC, Boca Raton.

Richards, R.S., Wang, L., & Jelinek, H. (2007). Erythrocyte oxidative damage in chronic fatigue syndrome. *Arch.Med.Res.*, 38, 94-98.

Schwartz, R.B., Komaroff, A.L., Garada, B.M., Gleit, M., Doolittle, T.H., Bates, D.W., Vasile, R.G., & Holman, B.L. (1994). SPECT imaging of the brain: comparison of findings in patients with chronic fatigue syndrome, AIDS dementia complex, and major unipolar depression. *AJR Am.J Roentgenol.*, 162, 943-951.

Shoemaker, R.C. & House, D.E. (2006). Sick building syndrome (SBS) and exposure to water-damaged buildings: time series study, clinical trial and mechanisms. *Neurotoxicol.Teratol.*, 28, 573-588.

Sperling, J.L.H. & Sperling, F.A.H. (2009). Lyme borreliosis in Canada: biologicaldiversity and diagnostic complexity from an entomological perspective. *Can.Entomol.*, 141, 521-549.

Straus, D.C. (2009). Molds, mycotoxins, and sick building syndrome. *Toxicol.Ind.Health.*, 25, 617-635.

Streeten, D.H. & Bell, D.S. (1998). Circulating blood volume in chronic fatigue syndrome. *Journal of Chronic Fatigue Syndrome*, 4.

Weingart, S.N., Wilson, R.M., Gibberd, R.W., & Harrison, B. (2000). Epidemiology of medical error. *BMJ*, 320, 774-777.

White, K.P. & Harth, M. (2001). Classification, epidemiology, and natural history of fibromyalgia. *Curr Pain Headache Rep.*, 5, 320-329.

Wojciechowska-Koszko, I., Maczynska, I., Szych, Z., & Giedrys-Kalemba, S. (2011). Serodiagnosis of borreliosis: indirect immunofluorescence assay, enzyme-linked immunosorbent assay and immunoblotting. *Arch.Immunol.Ther.Exp.(Warsz.).*, 59, 69-77.

Bonus Session

New and Future Directions

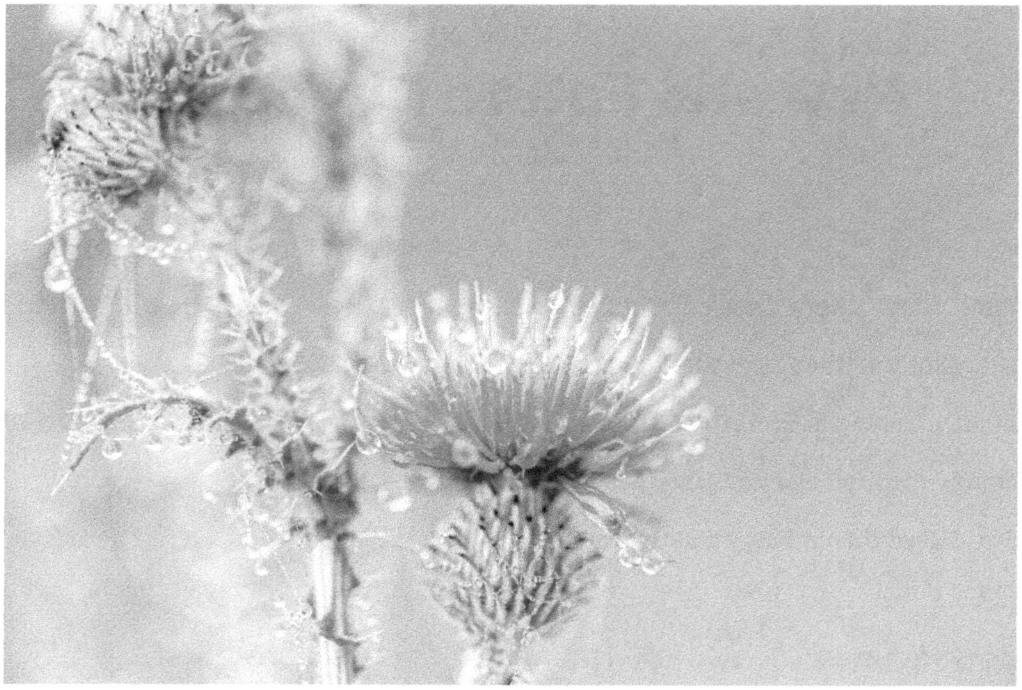

As Is

Seeing the world as it is
Takes courage
We like our veils and illusions.

Being who I am, as is
Takes everything I am
Requires a present focus
A loving eye
My own hand, soft
To my own cheek, wet.

Here I am, as is.

Carol Hechtenthal, Calgary, AB

Bonus Session

New and Future Directions

Introduction

This bonus chapter is all about hope. In it, I share emerging research that may be helpful, even transformational, for people with complex chronic diseases. I have been trying these strategies myself and continue to see improvements in my own health. I have been teaching these new ideas and strategies to my ***Live! with Dr. Stein*** community and people are reporting improvements. The contents of this chapter are evidence-based but have not yet been specifically studied in complex chronic diseases.

Why am I sharing information that hasn't undergone randomized controlled trials in ME, CFS, FM, ES and long COVID? Because I'm impatient. Although research is progressing and we are learning so much about what is going on at the cellular level, the research hasn't yet translated into effective treatments.

As we wait for effective disease-specific biomedical interventions, research in other fields is identifying self-management and biomedical strategies that improve health and longevity. I am hopeful that these strategies, though not curative, can benefit people with complex chronic diseases. In this bonus session, I am sharing a few of what I consider the most exciting developments.

The chapter starts with chronic inflammation, generally agreed to be at the core of most chronic diseases. Then I discuss four strategies to decrease inflammation: purposeful intermittent exposure to stressors, syncing one's biology with the sun, leveraging our quantum natures and rewiring the brain using neuroplasticity-based daily practice.

Although these topics may seem unrelated, they all tie into some of the body's most essential mechanisms of cellular repair. If we can turn on our repair machinery at regular intervals, we will live longer and healthier. Isn't that what we all want?

Chronic Inflammation: A Root Cause of Chronic Disease

Inflammation is an essential time-limited response of the immune system to defend against invaders and heal injury. Acute inflammation is usually obvious. You notice redness, swelling and heat in the inflamed area. And you typically have pain to encourage you to rest the area and let it heal.

Chronic inflammation occurs when the acute inflammation doesn't turn off as it should, either because the cause of the problem is still there, or because other (most often lifestyle-related) factors keep adding fuel to the inflammatory fire.

It might not be too strong a statement to say that virtually all chronic diseases are associated with chronic inflammation, including the big four: cancer, atherosclerotic heart disease, diabetes, and neurodegenerative diseases and things you might not expect, such as major depression. Chronic inflammation is found in all complex chronic diseases, such as ME, CFS, FM, long COVID, and chronic pain.

How do you know if you have chronic inflammation? In severe cases, you may have an elevated, highly sensitive C-reactive protein (hsCRP) test result. But many people with complex chronic diseases have inflammation, and their hsCRP is normal. There are private test panels measuring "hidden" inflammation, but they are expensive, and none are in widespread use.

What causes chronic inflammation? In this section, I mention a few of the most common treatable causes of chronic inflammation to give you a sense of some things you can do to decrease inflammation.

Caloric Overload

One of the most common causes of inflammation is taking in more calories than we need. This leads to the gain of subcutaneous fat (the outer, visible fat). When the fat cells on the outside of the body are too full to store any more fat, they release fat into the blood (triglycerides go up at this point), and that fat is stored in our essential organs, including the liver and pancreas. This is called visceral fat.

Visceral fat is inflammatory. It produces immune molecules that are a root cause of chronic inflammation. A FibroScan is a special ultrasound that measures the amount of fat in the liver and whether it has caused fibrosis. FibroScans are relatively easy to obtain.

The evidence-based treatments for inflammation caused by calorie overload include

- Either a very low-calorie diet (e.g., 800 cals/day) or intermittent fasting. Some of the most definitive research on this has been done at Newcastle University in the UK. They used an 800-calorie/day diet to achieve a lasting cure from diabetes for two years. After losing 15 kg, the participants were slowly put back on a maintenance diet and maintained the benefits. You can read more at https://www.ncl.ac.uk/magres/research/diabetes/reversal/#publicinformation.
- Minimize ultra-processed foods, including high-calorie foods, pre-packaged and ready-to-eat meals, processed bread and meat and most snacks. Any food packaged with chemical ingredients and a long shelf life is problematic (Tristan Asensi, Napoletano, Sofi, & Dinu, 2023).

- Eat more organic, colorful, whole plant-based foods.
- Support your microbiome with fiber-rich and fermented foods.

You might be wondering whether anti-inflammatory drugs will help with this kind of inflammation. They have been tested and don't decrease the hidden inflammation associated with chronic diseases. But some drugs used for diabetes, like SGLT2 inhibitors, GLP-1 agonists, DPP4 inhibitors, metformin and sulfonylureas decrease inflammation. We don't know if this is happening because of the effects on sugar levels, insulin levels and weight or because the drugs are acting directly on the immune system. Metformin, at least, seems to have direct anti-inflammatory effects.

Other important causes of chronic inflammation include poor dental health, chronic infection such as long COVID or chronic Lyme disease and chronic exposure to toxins like glyphosate or mold in water-damaged buildings. Each of these causes has special protocols for testing and treatment.

Hormesis: Using Intermittent Stressors to Improve Health

One of the ways we can lower inflammation is through a process called hormesis. Hormesis is our cells' ability to respond to intermittent low levels of stress by becoming more functional and resilient. Here is a common example. When we exercise, our muscles are slightly damaged. They respond to this by repairing and, in the process, become stronger. If the stress is too great, the muscles would be too severely damaged to recover. If the stress isn't enough, the muscles won't notice there is a problem and won't repair or strengthen.

If you consider how our distant ancestors lived, they were frequently exposed to changes in activity, food availability, temperature and sunlight. It makes sense that our bodies would have built-in mechanisms to thrive under these unstable conditions. We have evolved networks that sense what is going on in and around our bodies, and these networks control virtually all aspects of metabolism, energy production, cell function and even longevity (Calabrese et al., 2023). These are the superpowers of our cells. Common hormetic stressors include

- intermittent fasting,
- exposure to heat or cold, and
- exposure to red and infrared light.

These sensing networks are interconnected and constantly communicate with each other. They can be activated by any of the stressors I discuss here. We generally have the capacity to increase our cellular function by up to 30%. If we didn't, we wouldn't have survived our unpredictable environment. Hormesis works on our behalf throughout life. This means there is always the possibility of improvement.

Most people think that stressing our cells and bodies is bad and to be avoided. But this is not true. Cells need to be exposed to enough stressors of the right kind on a regular basis to function optimally (Nunn, Guy, & Bell, 2016).

Not all stressors are beneficial. Here are three key features of hormesis:

- The nature of the stressor. Some stressors are never beneficial at any dose. Examples include air pollution, methylmercury in fish, DDT on food, and BPA in plastics. We don't build resilience to these. Exposure to these toxins—especially exposures to multiple toxins at the same time, as is common in our modern world—causes serious health problems that cannot be overcome by hormesis.
- The amount (dose) of the stressor is vital. Hormetic stressors are typically beneficial at low doses but may be toxic or even fatal at higher doses. The key is to find the sweet spot, not too low, not too high. For example, if you are cold enough to shiver, this is a hormetic stressor. If you stay in the cold and develop hypothermia, you have overdone it, resulting in damage if you are unable to warm up safely.
- Hormetic stressors must be intermittent to be effective. Examples include alternating exercise with rest or eating with fasting. This is because the benefits of hormesis are not due to the stressor itself but rather to the cells' response to the stressor, and this response takes time.

Here are some evidence-based hormetic protocols.

Time-Restricted Eating (TRE)

Time-restricted eating is one of the most well-researched hormetic strategies. It refers to limiting when we eat to a window of time and then fasting long enough overnight for the repair networks to have time to do their job. We need to fast for at least 12 hours every night for benefits to occur, and if we fast for a bit longer, 14 – 16 hours, the benefits are greater.

The timing of the eating is also important. For the best effects, choose an eating window earlier in the day and maintain at least 3 hours between the last calorie intake and bedtime.

Cold Immersion

Believe it or not, cold immersion activates many of the same molecular pathways as other hormetic stressors, such as exercise and time-restricted eating. It turns out that athletes have been cold plunging for decades because cold immersion helps people recover faster from exercise and exertion. This includes people with ME and CFS who endure the 2-day CPET (cardiopulmonary exercise test).

A research-based cold immersion protocol is to immerse yourself up to the neck in cold water below 12°C (54°F) for up to 3 minutes. Stay in until you start to shiver for the best effect. Aim for a total of 11 minutes per week of cold immersion (Søberg, 2023).

Your own judgement is your best guide. If at first you are shivering unbearably after only a few seconds, stop there. Keep trying, knowing that cold immersion is a hormetic stressor that, in small, intermittent doses, will increase your tolerance over time, as well as your overall health as the cellular benefits accumulate.

Red and Infrared Light

When I first learned about the benefits of red and infrared light therapy in Dr. Norman Doidge's 2015 book *The Brain's Way of Healing* (Doidge, 2015), I didn't believe what I was reading. No one taught me in medical school that, like plants, we gain energy from the sun.

I started investigating and found there were thousands of peer-reviewed publications and over 300 meta-analyses (studies identifying trends among studies) concluding that red and infrared LED arrays and lasers (photobiomodulation) are effective in a wide variety of conditions. That was 10 years ago. Confirmatory research has continued to build. A recent meta-analysis of over 9000 participants concludes photobiomodulation benefits diverse conditions, including burning mouth syndrome, diabetic foot ulcers, head and neck pain, fibromyalgia and cognitive impairment (Son et al., 2025). What's better, no serious side effects have been reported when used as recommended.

Buoyed by that information, I bought a system and started offering photobiomodulation (light therapy) to patients. Many of them reported benefits to energy, sleep, pain and mood.

Here's how it works.

- Red and infrared wavelengths of light are absorbed by the mitochondria, our energy powerhouses. The absorbed energy (photons of light) activates cytochrome C oxidase, the final enzyme in the production of cellular energy (ATP).
- When the cells have more energy, they can spend it however they want and need to, including improved healing, an anti-inflammatory effect equal to that of diclofenac (a commonly used anti-inflammatory drug) and increased blood flow.
- This leads to faster and more complete healing from injury and surgery.
- The hormetic aspect of light therapy is that ATP production creates free radicals. This hormetic stressor causes the affected cells to increase their antioxidant capacity, thereby becoming stronger and more resilient against future oxidative stressors.

One of the best ways to get full-spectrum red and IR light is to go outside. The sun emits red and infrared light all year round, and you don't have to be in direct sunlight to benefit. In fact, sitting under a tree is one of the best ways to soak up the rays. Plants absorb green light and reflect and transmit the red and IR wavelengths. Getting outside for an hour a day can meet most of your needs. And there are additional benefits of being outside, like the production of the natural antioxidant melatonin when the skin is exposed to red and IR light. You do not benefit if you are inside next to a window since most glass reflects red and IR light in the name of energy efficiency.

If you are intent on spending some money, you can buy a device. Note that no device on the market is full-spectrum; most have up to 4 different wavelengths.

How to use a red/IR light array:

- You can choose a small device to treat areas of body pain or injury by directing the light to the area in question.
- You can use photobiomodulation for general health and overall energy by treating the head and neck. This energizes the blood passing through the neck, which then circulates around the body.
- There are experimental transcranial (through the skull) devices to treat brain disorders like depression and dementia.

I suggest doing your research before buying a red/IR light device. Make sure the amount of light emitted is clearly marked. Ask for third-party testing to ensure the power claims are valid. Remember, this is hormesis, so bigger is not necessarily better—hormesis requires the right dose at the right distance for the right amount of time. Use the panel only as directed, e.g., 15-30 minutes to affected areas. Remember that effective hormetic stress is intermittent—treating affected areas every other day is recommended.

To get the benefits of hormesis, you must start low and build up slowly. This cannot be emphasized enough. It takes time for cells to up their game. Just like a non-runner can't possibly run a marathon this week, a cell cannot operate at optimal capacity without adequate preparation.

Circadian Biology: Timing Is Everything

All living things, including humans, have an inner "clock." Actually, we have billions of them. Every organ, cell and gene has its own clock. Even the bacteria living in our colon have clocks. Our main body clock, also referred to as circadian rhythm, runs on a roughly 24-hour cycle. It regulates when we sleep, eat, feel alert, and even how our organs and immune system work.

Modern life—artificial lighting, irregular sleep, late-night eating and screen time—disconnects us from the Earth's natural rhythm. This can contribute to problems such as fatigue, poor sleep, digestive issues, inflammation, heart disease, diabetes, depression, lowered immunity and decreased cellular repair. When cells aren't in good working order, inflammation results (Martel, Ojcius, & Young, 2025).

How can we keep our body clock strong?

Exposure to Sunlight

Daily exposure to outdoor sunlight is the single most important thing you can do to stabilize and strengthen your circadian clock. Light is the number one zeitgeist (rhythm setter) in the body, and people who expose themselves to natural outdoor sunlight have lower rates of most chronic diseases. It is recommended to go outside first thing in the morning, during midday and at sunset for the best results.

Eating Schedule

After light exposure, the next most important signal to the body is the first meal of the day. When we eat in the morning, we let the body know it is time to wake up and burn the food just ingested to create the energy needed to fuel the day's activities. Our bodies expect food during the day, not late at night. Digestion takes several hours to complete. When we eat, our heart rate and blood pressure (BP) increase, and our body is aroused and awake. This isn't what we want at night. At night, we want the heart rate and BP to drop so that we are relaxed and can sleep soundly.

If we eat too late in the day, it will be harder to sleep, and the digestive organs will not work optimally because they are getting mixed messages: messages from the sun that it is time to rest and recover and messages from us that it is time to digest food and produce energy (Manoogian, Chow, Taub, Laferrere, & Panda, 2022). Compared with eating during the day, eating in the evening or at night is associated with

- slowed digestion and heartburn.
- elevated blood sugar and insulin.
- less effective cellular repair and recovery.
- imbalance of gut bacteria, increasing inflammation.

Time-restricted eating, discussed in the section on hormesis, strengthens our circadian biology and keeps digestive functions in sync. Limit eating to a 10–12-hour window (for example, 8 AM–6 PM) and stop eating at least 2–3 hours before bedtime. This gives the body time to rest and repair at night, including the all-important clearance of toxic garbage from the brain.

Activity Timing

Physical and mental activities send signals to the body clocks and strengthen circadian rhythm. Benefits of regular daytime activity include stronger bones, better joint health, sharper thinking, improved sleep, and better blood sugar control.

- Morning movement outdoors is especially powerful.
- Gentle activity after dinner helps manage blood sugar.
- Combining exercise with time-restricted eating may increase benefits.

Temperature

In ancestral times, humans were exposed to warm temperatures during the day and cooler temperatures at night. We can mimic this by taking a hot bath in the evening. After a bath, the body temperature drops, which enhances sleepiness. It is recommended to sleep in a room below 18 degrees C, even if you are under a duvet and only your face is exposed.

Quantum Biology-Inspired Health Strategies

For most of the past 120 years, since the birth of quantum physics, it has been assumed that there is a divide between tiny molecules, such as photons of light, that behave according to quantum laws, and larger organisms, like humans, that behave according to classical Newtonian laws. It has never been clear where the boundary is between quantum and classical objects, and as more research is done, that boundary is getting murkier. There has been a growing list of phenomena that classical physics can't explain, things like how birds return to the same place year after year during migration, how DNA replicates with so few errors but just enough to enable evolution to occur and how enzymes work so quickly and effortlessly to keep us alive.

For about 25 years, investigators have examined whether it is possible that our bodies have quantum properties, and the answer is increasingly YES (McFadden, 2016). The mitochondria have been studied more than most other organelles and are found to exhibit many quantum properties (Nunn et al., 2016).

There are fundamental aspects of quantum physics that explain important aspects of plant and animal biology:

- *Wave/particle duality*: The smallest particles in our bodies, electrons, protons and photons function both as particles and waves. When they act like waves, they exist as probability fields potentially being anywhere at any time. This quantum quality is critical for photosynthesis. It allows photons from the sun to get to the photosynthesis reaction centers quickly by the shortest route while maintaining close to 100% efficiency in energy production.

- *Coherence*: Particles can only behave in a quantum manner if there is coherence, meaning that everything in the environment is in sync. Quantum coherence can't occur in large areas like cells, but it can occur briefly in small parts of the cell that are temporarily tightly controlled, such as the electron transport chain in the mitochondria. Without coherence, the mitochondria would not be able to produce energy so efficiently.
- *Quantum tunneling*: Tunneling allows an electron or proton to move through a charged barrier despite not having the energy to do so. It is like rolling a stone up a hill. Quantum tunneling allows particles like electrons and protons to move against a huge hill of like charge and get to the other side like a ghost moving through a wall with ease. Quantum tunneling allows our DNA to mutate enough to adapt to new environments, but not so much to have runaway cancer. And it enables enzymes to work.
- *Quantum entanglement*: Particles like electrons and protons that were once in connection with each other remain in connection even after they are separated by great distances (like being on opposite sides of the universe). This is thought to explain how birds navigate so precisely during migration. Tiny changes in the Earth's magnetic field influence the entanglement of photons in birds' eyes, providing critical information for the birds to know which way to fly.

Are there ways we can optimize the quantum functions in our body? Yes, there are. Not surprisingly, these strategies all have to do with living an ancestral life. You are going to start seeing some common themes emerge.

Daily Exposure to Sunlight

In addition to the circadian benefits of exposing one's eyes to sunlight every day, we are discovering a long list of molecules in our bodies that act as chromophores, meaning they are responsive to specific wavelengths of light. It has even been shown that human molecules produce light and use it to communicate with other molecules.

- The morning balance of blue, red and IR wavelengths gets your body off to a healthy start by activating cortisol and other hormones.
- About one hour after sunrise, when the sun is about 10 degrees from the horizon, spend up to 20 minutes outside. Exposure to UVA light activates serotonin, dopamine and other important neurotransmitters so your brain can function properly. Could sunlight be a natural antidepressant?
- Mid-day is the best time to get exposure to UVB light, creating vitamin D in the skin.

What We Eat

What we eat is important. It is thought that information from light is stored in plants and communicates important information to the body about environmental conditions and the season of the year. If we don't eat locally, our bodies get conflicting information. It doesn't expect to gorge on fresh fruit in the middle of winter. Fruit was only available to our human ancestors in season. For this reason, quantum theorists suggest eating seasonal and local foods as much as possible. If you live in Canada or another northern clime, this means eating more meat and root vegetables in the winter and more greens and locally grown fruits in the summer.

Exclusion Zone Water

99% of the molecules in our body (67% by weight) are water. We take it for granted that every molecule of water is created equally. But this may not be true. There is increasing evidence that the water in our bodies is different from water in a glass, a lake or an ocean. The water in our bodies (in cells and next to membranes and proteins), when found next to hydrophilic (water-loving) surfaces, forms a distinct exclusion zone (EZ) that excludes certain molecules, including toxins (Pollack, 2013). EZ water is more like a gel than a liquid (the so-called 4th phase of water). One could think of it as protective. And it appears that infrared light helps maintain structured water in our bodies, yet another way in which IR light is essential for good health.

How do we get EZ water?

- The water produced by our mitochondria as a product of energy production is pure EZ water. Interestingly, we produce more mitochondrial water from fat than from protein or carbohydrate.
- Infrared light from the sun is the #1 strategy to build and maintain EZ water because it structures water directly and supports our mitochondria to create structured water. This is yet another reason to spend time outside during daylight hours.
- Structured water is said to exist in natural streams and vortexes.
- Toxins like glyphosate, heavy metals, and non-native EMF (Wi-Fi, blue light in the evening, LED light in the daytime) deplete EZ water. Minimize exposure to these toxins.
- Devices are sold that claim to structure water, but I have not come across convincing evidence of this.

Voltage

We are electric and have a body voltage just like a battery. Our body pH is slightly alkaline, 7.35–7.45. This means, in good health, our bodies have ample electrons, enough to create a negative charge in every cell. The lining of blood vessels needs to be negatively charged for the blood to flow easily around the body. Since negative charges repel each other, if all cells are negatively charged, everything can move with ease.

EZ (structured) water helps our body maintain a negative charge, and IR light helps structure the water. Everything in nature fits together. Electrons and protons are shuttled around the body to where they are needed by connective tissue called fascia. Insufficient electrons lead to inflammation, pain and stiffness.

How do we get and maintain enough electrons?

- As soon as you connect your bare skin with the Earth, electrons flow into the body and go where they are needed to establish the negative charge we need to function (Sinatra, Sinatra, Sinatra, & Chevalier, 2022). This is difficult to do in cold, icy climates.
- Consider buying grounding devices (e.g., grounding pads or sheets) to ground you when you are inside.

Mitochondrial Function

It is becoming increasingly apparent that impaired mitochondrial dysfunction underlies most chronic diseases (Wallace, 2005). To function optimally, mitochondria need an ample supply of electrons, red and infrared light and oxygen. Modern indoor living depletes these critical resources, leading to mitochondrial dysfunction, decreased energy production and then to inflammation and chronic disease. Here are some ways to support your mitochondria.

- Keep a regular schedule in sync with the sun.
- Prioritize daily exposure to sunlight (red and IR).
- Ground daily (touch your bare skin to the Earth) to keep the electrons flowing to your mitochondria.
- Minimize exposure to non-native electromagnetic radiation from high voltage power lines, dirty electricity, and wireless devices.
- Introduce some hormetic strategies (time-restricted eating, cold plunges, sauna, intermittent hypoxia, molecular hydrogen—they all strengthen mitochondrial function).
- Avoid toxins; they damage mitochondria and other important cellular components.

Neuroplasticity: Rewire Your Way to Better Health

Many people living with chronic illness experience symptoms such as pain, fatigue, brain fog, and heightened sensitivity to light, movement, sound and touch. These symptoms are real and often very disabling. Research shows that the brain itself plays a powerful role in generating certain symptoms and shaping how we experience them. This is due to neuroplasticity—the brain's ability to change its wiring and function in response to lived experience.

Neuroplasticity explains both why symptoms can persist and, most importantly, how they can improve. When we experience something noxious (painful, smelly, traumatic), the brain remembers it. And thereafter, under certain circumstances, such as the presence of fear or strong emotions, the brain can get stuck in this sensitive state. In fact, it can become more sensitive over time to experiences similar to the original trigger. This is called conditioning—neural circuits form to warn you that there is a problem.

Conditioning is helpful if there is a problem. It takes over to protect us without us having to think about it each time. But in the case of chronic symptoms, the original trigger or injury may be in the past, and the brain keeps generating symptoms to warn you of a problem that no longer exists. This is called central sensitization. Without some intervention on your part, you can become more and more sensitive and more symptomatic over time.

Not all symptoms are generated directly by the brain. If an elephant steps on your foot, there will be tissue damage, sending a strong message to your brain so that you will take protective action. How can you determine whether your symptoms are caused by neuroplasticity? Neuroplastic symptoms have certain characteristics that can tip you off that you have a problem with the brain rather than ongoing tissue damage. These signs include the following:

- Sensitivity to cold or ice or worsening of symptoms after repeated stimulation (like pressure, heat, or muscle contraction).
- Light touch feeling painful—even in areas that aren't normally sore.
- Increased irritability, low mood, or worsening of symptoms with stress, grief, anger, or fear.
- Heightened sensitivity to light, noise, touch, or smell.
- Clumsiness or less awareness of where your body is in space.
- Symptoms that shift around the body or change in nature.
- Feeling better with heat.
- Fatigue that is out of proportion to activity.
- Trouble with clear, quick thinking (brain fog).

If you recognize four or more of these signs, your brain's wiring is likely amplifying your symptoms. The same neuroplasticity that contributes to your symptoms can also be used for healing. Anything created by the brain can, with training, be reshaped by the brain. This section introduces you to a method to rewire your brain to become less sensitive to perceived danger signals.

The first law of neuroplasticity is sometimes described as *"What fires together, wires together."* This means that whatever we repeatedly think, feel, or do becomes hardwired in the brain. If we take charge of our daily experiences, we can reverse these changes and build the capacity for health.

Because of its physiologic properties, a neuron can't do two things at once. This means that if each time you experience a symptom, you redirect your attention towards experiences and activities that are uplifting, creative and connecting, you can override symptom generation and create or restore healthy neural circuits. This neuroplasticity-based approach is not about ignoring symptoms, but about gently guiding the brain toward new functional patterns.

Calm and Safety

Create a sense of calm, reassurance, and physical/emotional safety. Stress and fear keep the nervous system on high alert. Calm tells the brain the body is safe. When the brain judges that things are safe, it stops generating symptoms to get your attention. They can literally melt away.

Active Redirection

Each time you notice a symptom, treat it as a reminder to redirect your brain. Choose an activity that holds your attention, is enjoyable, or feels meaningful. Examples include the following:

- Gentle touch or self-massage
- Movement or exercise within your capacity
- Positive self-talk
- Visualization (e.g., imagining the brain cooling down)
- Empathy or connecting with loved ones
- Calming scents or sounds

Life Goals and Meaning

Focus not only on your symptoms but also on building the life you want. Notice, I don't say rebuilding because you may decide to make some changes. Align daily activities with your values and goals. This helps the brain form positive, health-oriented pathways.

Daily Practice

Like learning a musical instrument or a new language, retraining the brain takes practice. Spend about an hour a day, broken into small periods, on rewiring your brain. Practice calming, redirection, and life-focused strategies.

Every time you respond differently to your symptoms—choosing calm and redirection instead of worry or fear—you are teaching your brain new habits. Over time, these healthier habits grow stronger and old pain pathways weaken.

The bottom line is that you have agency. At any age and no matter how long you have been ill, if your symptoms have some of the neuroplastic features I mention above, your brain can be retrained. With gentle, consistent practice, it is possible to reduce symptoms and reclaim more of the life you want.

Bonus Session References

Calabrese, E. J., Osakabe, N., Di Paola, R., Siracusa, R., Fusco, R., D'Amico, R., . . . Calabrese, V. (2023). Hormesis defines the limits of lifespan. *Ageing Research Reviews, 91*, 102074. doi:https://dx.doi.org/10.1016/j.arr.2023.102074

Doidge, N. (2007). *The Brain that Changes Itself*: Penguin Books.

Doidge, N. (2015). *The Brain's Way of Healing*. New York: Viking.

Manoogian, E. N. C., Chow, L. S., Taub, P. R., Laferrere, B., & Panda, S. (2022). Time-restricted Eating for the Prevention and Management of Metabolic Diseases. *Endocrine Reviews, 43*(2), 405–436. doi:https://dx.doi.org/10.1210/endrev/bnab027

Martel, J., Ojcius, D. M., & Young, J. D. (2025). Circadian rhythmicity and human health. *Biomed J, 48*(3), 100855. doi:https://dx.doi.org/10.1016/j.bj.2025.100855

McFadden, J. A.-K. J. (2016). *Life on the Edge: The Coming of Age of Quantum Biology*: Black Swan.

Nunn, A. V., Guy, G. W., & Bell, J. D. (2016). The quantum mitochondrion and optimal health. *Biochem Soc Trans, 44*(4), 1101–1110. doi:https://dx.doi.org/10.1042/BST20160096

Pollack, G. H. (2013). *The Fourth Phase of Water: Beyond Solid, Liquid, and Vapor*: Ebner & Sons.

Sinatra, S., Sinatra, D., Sinatra, S., & Chevalier, G. (2022). Grounding – The Universal Anti-Inflammatory Remedy. *Biomedical Journal, 46*. doi:https://dx.doi.org/10.1016/j.bj.2022.12.002

Søberg, S. (2023). *Winter Swimming: The Nordic Way Towards a Healthier and Happier Life*: Quercus Publishing.

Son, Y., Lee, H., Yu, S., Kim, H. J., Park, J., Woo, S., . . . Yon, D. K. (2025). Effects of photobiomodulation on multiple health outcomes: an umbrella review of randomized clinical trials. *Systematic Reviews, 14*(1), 160. doi:https://dx.doi.org/10.1186/s13643-025-02902-3

Tristan Asensi, M., Napoletano, A., Sofi, F., & Dinu, M. (2023). Low-Grade Inflammation and Ultra-Processed Foods Consumption: A Review. *Nutrients, 15*(6). doi:https://dx.doi.org/10.3390/nu15061546

Wallace, D. C. (2005). A mitochondrial paradigm of metabolic and degenerative diseases, aging, and cancer: a dawn for evolutionary medicine. *Annual Review of Genetics, 39*, 359–407. doi:https://dx.doi.org/10.1146/annurev.genet.39.110304.095751

Charts and Tools

Karnofsky Energy Rating Scale adapted for use in ME/CFS

From Bell,D.S. (1995) *The Doctor's Guide to Chronic Fatigue Syndrome,* Boston, MA.

Further adapted by Dr. Ellie Stein

100% Totally well; no concerns about fatigue. You can think clearly and do several things at once. You can exercise to your maximum potential without any problems.

90% Energy good but you feel fatigued after hard exercise.

80% You feel well with respect to your energy but must monitor your energy through the day. Your thinking is good but not quite clear. Tasks are easy and you can still do multiple tasks at once. You are fatigued after moderate exercise. Full time work is possible for most.

70% Your overall energy is OK but everything you do is much more difficult and your energy is easily shifted. Your thought processes are much slower and more difficult and memory is poor. Exercise tolerance is poor and any strenuous exercise will make you feel unwell while light activity is tolerable. You can achieve a full day (8 hours) of tasks, but it requires a high degree of effort. You are too tired to do anything additional such as socializing. Full time work is possible only if you do not have to do any household tasks, errands or childcare. Part time work is possible for most.

60% You are able to complete 1/2 day of tasks and feel tired during it. Your thinking and memory are poor. You must rest at some point in the day. Even with rest, there is no part of the day in which you feel normal with respect to energy or can think clearly. Part time work is possible only if hours are flexible to coincide with your energy peaks and you do not have to do any household tasks, errands or childcare.

50% Your energy only allows you to do about 3 tasks per day (2-3 hours of activity). Your energy is easily drained. Thought processes are difficult. Your exercise tolerance is poor; walking up stairs is difficult.

40% You can only perform 2 light tasks per day. Physical exercise is not tolerable. Your thought processes are very slow and your memory is poor.

30% You can only perform one light task per day, any extra physical movement makes you feel unwell. You have difficulty reading and writing.

20% You are unable to perform any daily tasks; even going to the bathroom is tiring. The most physical exertion you can manage is to sit in a chair for short periods.
Emotions are very unstable and fluctuate without warning.

10% You are in bed for most of the day and you have zero tolerance for anything extra. You are frequently too exhausted to even eat.

Sleep Chart

Name ______________ **Date** ______________ **to** ______________
Meds:
Supplements:

Date	% Energy	Pain	Activities/other factors	Bed Time Meds	Initiate mins	Depth	Aware	wake #/min	deep/ light	Refresh -ment

Graph

% Fcn	Mon	Tue	Wed	Thurs	Fri	Sat	Sun	Mon	Tues	Wed	Thurs	Fri	Sat	Sun
95%														
85%														
75%														
65%														
55%														
45%														
35%														
25%														
15%														

Adapted from the "sleep sheet" of Dr. Beverley Tompkins, Burke Institute, Calgary

Use of the Sleep Chart

The sleep chart can be adapted to individual needs. The column headings can be changed to include the most important symptoms for you. The graph at the bottom can be narrowed to the range usually experienced.

Evening Charting - the first 5 columns are filled out each evening before bed rating the day that just passed and recording bed time medication if any.

- **Energy is rated from 0 - 100%** using the Karnofsky Rating scale adapted for use in ME/CFS.
- **Pain is rated from 0 - 10 with 0/10** being an absence of pain and 10/10 being unbearable "call 911 now" pain.
- **Activities/Other factors -** Is a place to record events that happened during the day which may impact energy, pain, sleep etc. This would include time spent in activity such as errands, yard work, cleaning, walking or other exercise, the occurrence of illness or migraine, environmental exposure or psychological stress. Some people use the back of the page to record these events in more detail
- **Bed Time Meds -** List all medications and supplements that you take before bed, especially list any that you are changing the dose or timing of to see if it helps or impairs your sleep.

Morning Charting - The last 6 columns to the right of the bolded line are completed upon rising. They refer to the night that just passed.

- **Initiate minutes** - Estimate the number of minutes it took you to fall asleep
- **Depth** - Rated from 1 - 5 - where 1/5 is barely asleep and 5/5 is deep, uninterrupted, unaware, refreshing sleep
- **Aware** - Note the things you were aware of when you were supposed to be asleep

T - Temperature	1/2 - feeling 1/2 awake and 1/2 asleep

- **Wake #/min** - Estimate the number of times you woke up and the number of minutes you were awake during the night. e.g. if you woke 3 times for 1/2 hour each time you would put 3/90
- **Deep/Light** - Estimate the number of hours of deep sleep and the number of hours of light sleep, e.g. 2/6
- **Refreshment** - Morning refreshment is rated on a scale

H - Horrible	G - Good
P - Poor VG	VG - Very good
F - Fair	E - Excellent

Graph - At the end of the charting period plot all numerical variables on the graph below. You may convert a 1-10 pain scale to percentages if you wish. You may add pedometer steps or exercise durations to the columns. By adding up arrows for improved energy through the day or down arrows for decreased energy through the day you can judge if your energy expenditure is appropriate.

Adapted from the “sleep sheet” of Dr. Beverley Tompkins, Burke Institute, Calgary

Activity Log

Name: ______________________________ Date: ______________

Day	Monday	Tuesday	Wednesday	Thursday	Friday	Saturday	Sunday
No. of Hrs. Sleep 1:00 am – 8:00 am							
Sleep Quality		*1 = very poor*	*2 = poor*	*3 = fair*	*4 = good*	*5 = very good*	
Functional Capacity Scale at beginning of day							
0 – 10 (see reverse)							
Activities (please specify)							
8:00 am							
9:00 am							
10:00 am							
11:00 am							
12:00 pm							
1:00 pm							
2:00 pm							
3:00 pm							
4:00 pm							
5:00 pm							
6:00 pm							
7:00 pm							
8:00 pm							
9:00 pm							
10:00 pm							
11:00 pm							
12:00 am							
1:00 am							
No. of Mins. Walked / Day							
No. of Usable Hours / Day							
Functional Capacity Scale at end of day							
0 – 10 (see reverse)							

YOUR ACTIVITY LOG:

- Keep it in a handy place.
- Complete it every day.
- Take your completed logs to your doctor/other health care provider at follow-up visits.
- Your logs assist your doctor/other health care provider to adjust your treatment plan as needed.
- Completed logs may reassure your insurance company of your active ongoing participation in your treatment.

COMPLETING YOUR ACTIVITY LOG:

- You may change the times on the left hand side of the log to suit your usual schedule (e.g. if you usually get up at 10:00 am and go to bed at 2:00 am, write 10:00 am in as the first time, and adjust the other times accordingly).
- Please note your activities with one or two word(s) in the appropriate time slots (e.g. dressed, made bed, nap).

FUNCTIONAL CAPACITY SCALE:

- The Functional Capacity Scale incorporates energy rating, symptom severity, and activity level. The description after each scale number should help you to rate your functional capacity at the beginning and end of each day.

  0 = No energy, severe symptoms including very poor concentration; bed ridden all day; cannot do self-care (e.g. need bed bath to be given).

  1 = 10% energy, severe symptoms at rest, including very poor concentration; in bed most of the day; need assistance with self-care activities (e.g. tub bath).

  2 = 20% energy, severe symptoms at rest, including poor concentration; frequent rests or naps; need some assistance with limited self-care activities.

  3 = 30% energy, moderate symptoms at rest, including poor concentration; need frequent rests or naps; can do independent self-care but have severe post exertion fatigue.

  4 = 40% energy, moderate symptoms at rest, including some difficulty concentrating; need frequent rests throughout the day; can do independent self-care and limited activities of daily living (e.g. light housework, laundry); can walk for a few minutes per day.

  5 = 50% energy, mild symptoms at rest with fairly good concentration; need a.m. and p.m. rest; can do independent self- care and moderate activities of daily living, but have slight post exertion fatigue; can walk 10 – 20 minutes per day.

6 = 60% energy, mild or no symptoms at rest with fairly good concentration; need afternoon rest; can do most activities of daily living except vacuuming; can walk 20 – 30 minutes per day; can do volunteer work — maximum total time 4 hours per week, with flexible hours.

7 = 70% energy, mild or no symptom at rest with good concentration; can do more intense activities of daily living (e.g. grocery shopping, vacuuming) but may get post exertion fatigue if 'overdo'; can walk 30 minutes per day; can work limited hours, less than 25 hours per week; no or minimal social life.

8 = 80% energy, mild intermittent symptoms with good concentration; can do full self-care, work 40 hours per week, enjoy a social life, do moderate vigorous exercise three times per week.

9 = 90% energy, no symptoms with very good concentration, full work and social life; can do vigorous exercise three to five times a week.

10 = 100% energy, no symptoms, excellent concentration, over achiever (sometimes may require less sleep than average person).

NUMBER OF USABLE HOURS / DAY = Number of hours NOT asleep or resting/meditating with eyes closed

Environmental Health Clinic
Sunnybrook & Women's College Health Sciences Centre
Print design: Helen Kwan

Daily Diet Diary

Date____________________			Name_____________________				
Time	Food	Contents	Amount	Protein	Fat	Carbs	Cals
				Protein	Fat	Carbs	Cals
Total							
“servingsfruits_____		(1 serving = 1/2 cup)		complete protein _______			
“servingsveg _____				litres water ________			

Activity and Symptoms Chart

Name:____________________ Date ____________________ to ____________________

Date & Time	Activity	Symptom

Sleep Chart Adapted for Mood

Name ________________ Date __________________ to _____________________

Meds:

Supps:

Date	% Energy	Pain	Mood	Activities/other factors

% Fcn	Mon	Tue	Wed	Th	Fri	Sat	Sun	Mon	Tues	Wed	Th	Fri	Sat	Sun
95%														
85%														
75%														
65%														
55%														
45%														
35%														
25%														
15%														

www.ingramcontent.com/pod-product-compliance
Lightning Source LLC
LaVergne TN
LVHW060028210926
848481LV00013B/3816
* 9 7 8 0 9 8 8 1 5 1 0 2 4 *